Teen Health

Course 3

Student Activities Workbook

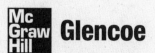
McGraw Hill Glencoe

New York, New York   Columbus, Ohio   Chicago, Illinois   Peoria, Illinois   Woodland Hills, California

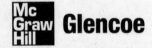

Glencoe

The McGraw·Hill Companies

Send all inquiries to:
Glencoe/McGraw-Hill
21600 Oxnard Street, Suite 500
Woodland Hills, CA 91367

ISBN 0-07-826186-4 (Student Edition)
ISBN 0-07-826187-2 (Teacher Annotated Edition)

10 11 12 13 14   009   13 12 11 10 09

Table of Contents

Introduction

This Workbook contains Study Guides, Activities, and Health Inventories to accompany the chapters in your student textbook.

The Study Guides are to be completed as you read each lesson. They will help you check your understanding of lesson content. Each Study Guide consists of approximately 15 items. The items outline the main ideas in the chapter. After you have completed all the items, you can use the Study Guide to review the information in the chapter as a whole.

Following each Study Guide, there are Activities—one for each lesson in your textbook. The Activities give you opportunities to apply your knowledge and practice health-related skills. A variety of formats is offered, including fill-in, short-answer, matching, classifying, and sequencing. In some Activities, you are asked to complete a table after reading a short passage or to label or number items on a diagram. Still other Activities involve writing short paragraphs, essays, or letters.

A Health Inventory follows the Activities for each chapter. Each Health Inventory offers you an opportunity to assess a particular aspect of your own health. A typical Health Inventory consists of 15 statements for which you are asked to indicate *yes* if the statement describes you or *no* if it does not or to indicate whether the statement describes you *always*, *sometimes*, or *never* (or *always*, *usually*, or *sometimes*). A few of the Health Inventories take the form of checklists in which you are asked to check the items that describe you. The purpose of the Health Inventories is to help you recognize what you are doing that is good for your health and identify behaviors that you need to change.

Chapter 1 Study Guide

> ## STUDY TIPS
> ✔ Read the chapter objectives.
> ✔ Look up any unfamiliar words.
> ✔ Read the questions below before you read the chapter.

   As you read the chapter, answer the following questions. Later you can use this guide to review the information in the chapter.

Lesson 1

1. Define *health*.

   _____

2. Identify the three sides of the health triangle, and list two aspects of each side.

   _____

   _____

   _____

   _____

   _____

3. Why is it important to work on keeping your health triangle balanced?

   _____

   _____

4. Explain why wellness is more than just being healthy.

   _____

   _____

   _____

Lesson 2

5. Identify three characteristics of adolescence.

_____

_____

_____

6. Define _hormones_.

_____

7. List two changes that occur during adolescence for each of the following: physical growth, mental and emotional growth, social growth.

_____

_____

_____

_____

_____

Lesson 3

8. Define _lifestyle factors_, and identify three positive lifestyle factors.

_____

_____

_____

9. Define _risk behavior_.

_____

10. Explain why abstinence from risk behavior is a wise choice for teens.

_____

_____

11. List two factors involved in taking responsibility for your health.

_____

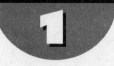

Activity 1

Use with Chapter 1, Lesson 1.

Applying Health Skills

Healthful Habits

Look at the statements below. In the space at the left of each statement, identify the side of the health triangle each behavior belongs to. Write *P* for physical, *M* for mental/emotional, or *S* for social. Then change any unhealthful behavior to a healthful one on the line beneath the statement.

_____ 1. going to a football game with friends

_____

_____ 2. eating plenty of fruits and vegetables

_____

_____ 3. hiding angry feelings

_____

_____ 4. helping a friend with a problem

_____

_____ 5. showing sadness when someone you care about dies

_____

_____ 6. staying up late every night

_____

_____ 7. quitting an activity and arguing when you do not get your way

_____

_____ 8. thinking that there isn't anything you do well

_____

Activity 2

Applying Health Skills

Changes During Adolescence

As individuals reach adolescence, they grow and change in ways that affect all three sides of the health triangle. These changes signal that the person is on the way to becoming an adult. Fill in the blanks below with the types of growth and change that occur during adolescence for each part of the health triangle. One answer has already been given for each of the three areas.

Physical Growth

Boys' voices grow deeper.

_____

_____

_____

Mental and Emotional Growth

You are able to solve increasingly complex problems.

_____

_____

_____

Social Growth

Finding new ways to relate to your family.

_____

_____

_____

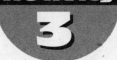

Applying Health Skills

Can You Control Your Health?

Read the following paragraphs about Sara and José. Then answer the questions that follow.

Sara and José are next-door neighbors. Although they have been friends for a long time, they are quite different. José is overweight. He has few friends and spends most of his free time watching television. He also likes computers, and he often stays up very late playing video games and surfing the Internet. José does not smoke, but his parents and some of his friends do. José has made some changes in his diet recently. He is avoiding foods high in salt and fat, and he's eating smaller portions and more fruits and vegetables. José likes to eat at Sara's house because her family is very health conscious and they eat nutritious foods.

Sara is slim. One of the most popular girls in the seventh grade, she has lots of friends. Sara spends much of her time on after-school activities, socializing with friends, practicing the flute, and studying. Despite a busy schedule, she makes sure that she gets at least eight hours of sleep every night. Sara goes bicycling nearly every day. Although she is very health conscious, Sara smokes sometimes, and often she does not wear a seat belt. José, on the other hand, always wears his seat belt because one of his friends was killed in a motor vehicle crash.

1. List one positive lifestyle factor for José and one for Sara.

_____

_____

_____

2. Identify one risk behavior for José and one for Sara.

_____

_____

_____

3. List two healthful decisions José has made.

_____

_____

4. Identify one precaution that José takes and one way that he practices abstinence to avoid serious health problems.

_____

Chapter 1 Health Inventory

A Totally Healthy You

Read the statements below. In the space at the left, write *yes* if the statement describes you, or *no* if it does not describe you.

_____ **1.** I seldom feel tired or run-down.

_____ **2.** I ask for help when I need it.

_____ **3.** I feel comfortable meeting people.

_____ **4.** I get at least eight hours of sleep each night.

_____ **5.** I can name at least three activities I perform well.

_____ **6.** I have at least one or two close friends.

_____ **7.** I can accept differences in people.

_____ **8.** I do 20 minutes or more of vigorous physical activity at least three times a week.

_____ **9.** I can express my feelings to others in healthy ways.

_____ **10.** I am happy most of the time.

_____ **11.** I can accept constructive criticism.

_____ **12.** I can accept other people's ideas and suggestions.

_____ **13.** I eat nutritious foods.

_____ **14.** I stay within 5 pounds of my appropriate weight range.

_____ **15.** I can say no to my friends if they are doing something I don't want to do.

Score yourself:

Write the number of *yes* answers here.

12–15: Your health practices are very good.

8–11: Your health practices are good.

5–7: Your health practices are fair.

Fewer than 5: You need to make some changes in your life.

Chapter 2 Study Guide

STUDY TIPS
- ✔ Read the chapter objectives.
- ✔ Look up any unfamiliar words.
- ✔ Read the questions below before you read the chapter.

As you read the chapter, answer the following questions. Later you can use this guide to review the information in the chapter.

Lesson 1

1. Define *decision making* and explain the value of decision-making skills.

_____

_____

2. Name the six steps in the decision-making process.

_____

_____

3. Define *goal setting*, and explain the benefit of goal-setting skills.

_____

_____

Lesson 2

4. Define *interpersonal communication*, and explain what it involves.

_____

_____

5. List four tips for improving speaking skills.

_____

_____

6. Name four ways to improve listening skills.

_____

_____

7. Identify four refusal skills.

_____

Lesson 3

8. Explain how stress can be positive.

_____

_____

9. Define *fight-or-flight response*, and explain how too much stress can affect the body.

_____

_____

_____

10. Name four stress management skills.

_____

Lesson 4

11. Identify three basic health skills.

_____

_____

12. Explain why a support system is important, and list some of the people it might include.

_____

_____

_____

13. List two internal influences and two external influences that can affect your health.

_____

_____

Activity 4

Applying Health Skills

Making Decisions

Making a decision can be difficult—especially if you are faced with a choice of two options that would have both positive and negative results. Using the decision-making process to think through the choices often helps. For each situation, write ideas to show what a person might think about in deciding what to do.

Situation 1

Lisa has been offered a part-time job after school. Her parents believe that school should be most important in a young person's life. However, Lisa could save her parents' money if she bought her own clothes.

1. What are Lisa's two options?

_____

2. What would be the positive results of each option?

_____

3. What would be the negative results of each option?

_____

_____

Situation 2

Barry has been invited to a party given by a popular older student. If he goes, Barry might be part of a popular group. However, liquor may be served, and Barry's family is strongly against drinking. Also, Barry's basketball coach is strict about his players avoiding alcohol.

4. What are Barry's two options?

_____

5. What would be the positive results of each option?

_____

6. What would be the negative results of each option?

_____

_____

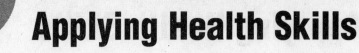

Activity 5

Applying Health Skills

What Did You Really Mean to Say?

Speaking is a small part of communication. Tone of voice and body language also deliver much of your message. Body language includes facial expressions, body movements, and gestures.

Complete the chart below by listing the facial expression and body language suitable to each situation. The first item has been done for you.

Situation	Facial Expression	Body Language
1. A friend's pet has died.	sad, sympathetic	
2. Your sister has made the field hockey team.		
3. Your friend is in trouble.		
4. Your parents have just punished you.		

Look at the pictures below. On the line following each, write what the picture communicates about the person.

5. _____

_____

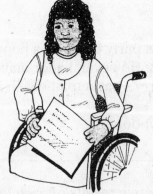

6. _____

_____

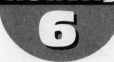

Activity 6 — Applying Health Skills

Managing Stress

Stress is the body's response to change. Anything that causes stress is called a stressor. Read each situation below. Identify the stressors in each case and then recommend an alternative course of action that may help reduce stress.

Situation	Stressors	Alternative Course of Action
1. Bev moved to a new school in the middle of the year. She had a difficult time catching up in her history class and got a D on her report card.		
2. Jodie has been so busy that she put off starting her English paper until the night before it is due. Now she's in a panic and doesn't know where to start.		
3. After Frank stopped wrestling, he quickly gained 20 pounds. The weight gain bothers him, and he thinks that it will hurt his chance of getting the lead in the school play.		
4. Mark got Saturday detention for being late to school. He admits that he has been staying up late because he is upset about his parents' recent divorce.		

Applying Health Skills

Finding the Information You Need

Accessing reliable health information will help you make wise decisions. Select and write the letter of the source from the list at the right that would most likely provide reliable information on each of the following. Each letter should be used only once.

_____ 1. Symptoms and treatment of lung cancer

_____ 2. Latest fad diets

_____ 3. Recent outbreak of flu in Europe

_____ 4. Immunizations you received as a child

_____ 5. Major airplane crash that occurred this morning

_____ 6. Number of cancer deaths in the United States in 1999

_____ 7. Link between obesity and heart disease

_____ 8. List of food additives allowed by law

_____ 9. Effect of aerobic exercise on the heart

_____ 10. Safety devices for the home

_____ 11. Incidence of Lyme disease in your community

_____ 12. Use of hypnosis for treating addiction

_____ 13. Programs to reduce alcohol-related car crashes among teens

_____ 14. Symptoms and treatment for chicken pox

_____ 15. Taking a course in CPR (cardiopulmonary resuscitation)

a. U.S. Centers for Disease Control and Prevention
b. County Board of Health
c. American Heart Association
d. *Encyclopedia of Diseases*
e. *Aerobic Exercise and Your Health* (book)
f. American Cancer Society
g. Television or radio news
h. Parents or guardians
i. World Health Organization
j. Web site on the Internet
k. *Psychology Today* (magazine)
l. Food and Drug Administration
m. American Red Cross
n. Mothers Against Drunk Driving
o. National Center for Injury Prevention and Control

Chapter **2** Health Inventory

Building a Good Foundation of Health Skills

Read each statement below. Decide how it describes your behavior. Write *always*, *sometimes*, or *never* in the space at the left of each statement.

_____ **1.** I weigh the possible outcomes of my decisions.

_____ **2.** I consider my values when I make decisions.

_____ **3.** I set goals for myself.

_____ **4.** I make plans for how to achieve my goals.

_____ **5.** I seek help and support from others when I set goals.

_____ **6.** I evaluate my progress toward reaching my goals.

_____ **7.** I use "I" messages when I express an opinion.

_____ **8.** I speak clearly when I communicate with others.

_____ **9.** I use refusal skills to help me say no effectively.

_____ **10.** I use relaxation techniques when I feel stressed.

_____ **11.** I try to keep a positive outlook when I'm under stress.

_____ **12.** I keep physically active.

_____ **13.** I set priorities to help manage my schedule.

_____ **14.** I consider the source of any health information I gather.

_____ **15.** I learn as much as possible about my health and health issues that may affect me.

Score yourself.

Give yourself 3 points for each *always* answer, 1 point for each *sometimes*, and 0 for each *never.* Write your score here.

36–45: Very good

26–36: Good

16–26: Room for improvement

Fewer than 16: Take a close look at your behavior, and see what changes you can make.

Chapter 3 Study Guide

STUDY TIPS

✔ Read the chapter objectives.

✔ Look up any unfamiliar words.

✔ Read the questions below before you read the chapter.

As you read the chapter, answer the following questions. Later you can use this guide to review the information in the chapter.

Lesson 1

1. Name three characteristics of an informed consumer.

_____

_____

2. List two internal and two external factors that influence your buying decisions.

_____

_____

3. Name four techniques that advertisers use to make their products or services appealing to consumers.

_____

_____

4. Describe three factors you should consider in comparison shopping.

_____

_____

5. Identify four of your basic rights as a consumer.

_____

_____

Lesson 2

6. List the two main roles of health care.

_____

7. Name four types of health care facilities available in most communities.

_____

_____

8. Define *health insurance*, and list three types of private insurance plans.

_____

_____

_____

Lesson 3

9. Define *health fraud*, and identify three signs to watch for to protect yourself from fraud.

_____

_____

_____

_____

_____

10. Name three types of consumer groups that can help consumers get satisfaction concerning defective products or services.

_____

_____

Lesson 4

11. Name two federal agencies that work to protect and enforce consumer rights.

_____

_____

12. Identify three tasks performed by local health departments.

_____

_____

_____

ACTIVITY 8

Applying Health Skills

Why Did You Buy That?

Your buying decisions are influenced by a variety of factors. Some are internal factors, such as personal taste, physical traits, or tradition. Other factors are external, including the influences of family, cost, advertising, the media, peers, and salespeople. Match each of the buying decisions below with the letter of the factor that influenced it. Some of the letters may be used more than once.

a. tradition
b. personal taste
c. physical traits
d. family
e. cost
f. media advertising
g. media
h. peers
i. salespeople

_____ 1. George saw a television commercial for a new brand of toothpaste gel with special whitening agents and decided to try it.

_____ 2. After trying on at least ten different pairs of jeans, Amy bought the most expensive pair because she thought she looked better in them than in the others.

_____ 3. The woman at the perfume counter convinced Maria to buy a new scent when she said that many young women were using it now.

_____ 4. Although the salesperson told John about a new cereal, he bought the brand he always buys.

_____ 5. Joan tried a new brand of laundry detergent because of her mother's recommendation.

_____ 6. After Matt read an article in a magazine about the nutritional benefits of soy, he switched from using regular milk to using soy milk on his cereal.

_____ 7. Becky always buys one particular brand of shoes because of the arch support they provide for her feet.

_____ 8. It took only a little prodding from his friends to convince Jake to buy the same style jacket as they wore.

_____ 9. Since Katy was on a tight budget, she bought the least expensive cat food she could find in the store.

_____ 10. Blue is Brandon's favorite color, and many of his clothes are blue.

_____ 11. Carey was undecided about which television to buy until she talked with her father, who usually gives her very good advice.

_____ 12. The infomercial on television really appealed to Vincent, and he decided to call and order the exercise equipment he saw on it.

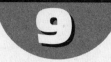

Applying Health Skills

Choosing Health Services

Write the correct title from the list below on each numbered answer line.

Titles:
> The Role of Health Care
> Types of Health Insurance
> Health Care Services for Teens
> People Who Provide Health Care
> Where Health Care Is Available
> Trends in Health Care

1. _____

primary care physicians
nurse practitioners
specialists

2. _____

health maintenance organizations (HMOs)
preferred provider organizations (PPOs)
point of service plans (POS's)

3. _____

private practices
clinics
hospitals

4. _____

prevent disease or injury from happening or getting worse
treat sickness or injury

5. _____

immunizations
skin care
sports exams

6. _____

birthing centers
hospices
telemedicine

Activity 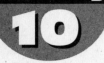 Applying Health Skills

The Biocaps Fraud

Assume that you are a consumer advocate investigating misleading advertisements. Look closely at the advertisement below. Then answer the questions on the lines provided.

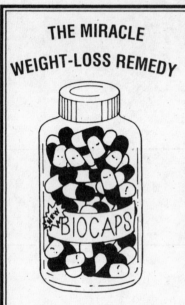

THE MIRACLE WEIGHT-LOSS REMEDY

Lose weight now, so you can enjoy the happy, carefree life you would like to lead. All-new **Biocaps** are the safe, scientific way to melt fat away overnight. **Biocaps** are based on an amazing new discovery. They boost the body's fat-burning rate and suppress your appetite without inconveniencing you in any way. Health care professional Sally DeVoto recommends **Biocaps!**

Everybody's trying this amazing new product. Simply eat as you usually do. There is no need to cut out your favorite fatty foods. Our special ingredient, Bioxen, is an extract from a South American shrub that has been found to be highly effective in strengthening the heart, curing cancer, and preventing colds, as well as quickly and easily melting fat away—with no exercise required and absolutely no risk to you. Simply take one capsule every hour, and watch your fat melt away. **Biocaps** are free of impurities such as the bacteria, insect parts, and mold found in competing products. Completely safe!

Order now! Send check or money order to:
Box 427, Sheldon, Iowa 51004

1. Which part of this advertisement do you consider most unbelievable?

_____

_____

Why?

_____

2. Which part of the advertisement provides a testimonial?

_____

3. Which part of the advertisement suggests that users will have a better lifestyle?

_____

_____

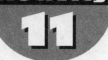

Activity 11

Use with Chapter 3, Lesson 4.

Applying Health Skills

Guarding the Public Health

Imagine that you are a volunteer for a community telephone service that directs callers to agencies, groups, and services for health information. Select and write the letter of the agency, group, or law from the list at the right that might help each caller below.

_____ 1. "I would like some information on the warning signs of a heart attack."

_____ 2. "Where can I find information about current research projects on AIDS?"

_____ 3. "Can you tell me if that car safety seat is still being manufactured? I heard there might be some problems with it."

_____ 4. "A pain reliever gave me stomach pains. There was no warning on the label."

_____ 5. "Where can I learn about different substance abuse prevention programs?"

_____ 6. "Whom can I contact about the recent outbreak of measles in my state?"

_____ 7. "I would like to take a swimmer's lifesaving course."

_____ 8. "There's a lot of garbage behind the hotel in our town. It's been there for more than a week."

_____ 9. "My son has started smoking. I'd like information on smoking and cancer."

_____ 10. "I earn very little income and have no health insurance. I was hoping to get some help getting access to some basic health services."

a. American Red Cross

b. State Health Department

c. Food and Drug Administration

d. American Heart Association

e. Substance Abuse and Mental Health Services Administration

f. Centers for Disease Control and Prevention

g. American Cancer Society

h. National Institutes of Health

i. Health Resources and Services Administration

j. Consumer Product Safety Commission

Chapter 3 Health Inventory

Are You a Wise Consumer?

Read the questions below. In the space at the left, write *yes* if the item describes you, or *no* if it does not describe you.

1. Do you know your rights as a consumer?

2. Do you compare products before you buy?

3. Are you aware of whether you are buying something because you *need* it or *want* it?

4. Do you read product labels before you buy something?

5. Are you aware of the influence of advertisements or friends when you make a purchase?

6. Do you know how to return an unsatisfactory or defective product?

7. Do you check an item to be sure that it works before you buy it?

8. Can you distinguish between facts and gimmicks in an advertisement?

9. Can you deal with a high-powered, pushy salesperson?

10. Do you ask the salesperson questions about an item you are thinking of buying?

11. Do you know where to get help with a consumer problem?

12. Do you know which medical problems are treated by which medical specialists?

13. Are you familiar with the health services that are available in your community?

14. Do you avoid being talked into purchases because they are "on sale"?

15. Do you care about getting the best product for your money?

Score yourself:

Write the number of yes answers here.

12–15: You are an alert consumer.

8–11: Pretty good; you're on the right track.

Fewer than 8: Buyers beware! Remember, it is your money and your health.

Chapter 4 Study Guide

STUDY TIPS
- ✔ Read the chapter objectives.
- ✔ Look up any unfamiliar words.
- ✔ Read the questions below before you read the chapter.

As you read the chapter, answer the following questions. Later you can use this guide to review the information in the chapter.

Lesson 1

1. Identify three abilities that define good mental and emotional health.

_____

_____

2. Define *personality*.

_____

_____

3. List four skills for improving self-esteem and your overall level of mental and emotional health.

_____

_____

Lesson 2

4. Identify three positive emotions.

_____

5. Define *emotional needs*, and name three basic emotional needs.

_____

_____

Lesson 3

6. Define *anxiety disorder*, and identify the five basic categories of these disorders.

_____

_____

7. Explain the difference between schizophrenia and clinical depression.

_____

_____

8. List three warning signs of suicide.

_____

_____

_____

Lesson 4

9. Describe the differences between the two main types of treatment for mental health problems.

_____

_____

_____

10. List some sources of help with mental and emotional problems.

_____

_____

Lesson 5

11. Name the five stages in the acceptance of dying.

_____

12. Name and describe the five stages of grief.

_____

_____

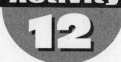

Applying Health Skills

The Road to Mental and Emotional Health

There are behaviors you can practice that will improve your self-esteem and your overall level of mental and emotional health. Read the situations described below, and recommend an action each person could take to build self-esteem and improve his or her mental and emotional health. Then look at the list of behaviors. Choose the behavior(s) each recommendation best demonstrates. Write the appropriate letters in the space provided.

Behaviors

a. motivate yourself

b. focus on strengths

c. understand and manage feelings

d. develop a positive attitude

e. learn from your mistakes

Situation 1

The day before a big basketball game, Lucy snaps at her brother. Lucy then recognizes that she is nervous about the big game.

Recommended Action:

_____

Behavior: _____

Situation 2

Lee hopes to play jazz trombone professionally one day. Tryouts for the school band are coming up. Lee is nervous because she knows that she will have to compete with older, more experienced students. However, Lee believes that she is a good musician.

Recommended Action:

_____

_____

Behavior: _____

Situation 3

Benji left his personal stereo next to an open window. It was ruined by a heavy rainfall. Benji's father points out that he should always close his window before going out.

Recommended Action:

_____

Behavior: _____

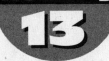

Applying Health Skills

Positive Messages

Read the statements below. Some show that the speaker has high self-esteem; others show low self-esteem. Classify each statement by writing *high* or *low* in the space at the left. On the line following each statement you have identified as low, rewrite the statement in a positive way.

_____ 1. "I didn't win the race, but I did my best time ever."

_____

_____ 2. "I'm not going to try out for the school choir because I know I won't get chosen."

_____

_____ 3. "There's no sense studying for the science test. I'm too dumb to pass it."

_____

_____ 4. "I'm so clumsy sometimes—maybe a dance class would help."

_____

_____ 5. "I'd like to ask Felicia to go skating with me, but I'm sure she'll say no."

_____

_____ 6. "I think I'll write a letter to Grandma. I'm sure she enjoys hearing from me."

_____

_____ 7. "I'd like to earn some money baby-sitting, but I don't know what to do with young children."

_____

_____ 8. "That art class sounds like fun, but I can't even draw a straight line."

_____

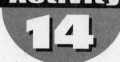 **Activity 14** **Applying Health Skills**

Emotional Needs and Abstinence

We all have basic emotional needs: the need to *feel worthwhile*, the need to *love and be loved*, and the need to *belong*. In addition, we all feel a variety of emotions every single day.

   Look at the emotions listed at the right. Read each quote. In the space after each quote, write the letter of the emotion that the quote expresses. Then write which of the three basic emotional needs described above is also expressed in each quote. Some quotes express more than one emotional need.

Quotes

Emotions
a. anger
b. love
c. fear
d. jealousy
e. happiness

1. "Should I ask Jackie to the dance? What if she says no?"

_____

2. "I can't wait to spend the holiday with my grandparents!"

_____

3. "Yes! I made the team!"

_____

4. "I get good grades, but I'm not as smart as my other friends."

_____

5. "My horrible little brother read my diary and found out what boys I like!"

_____

   Give reasons for abstaining from the behavior in each situation described below, and suggest a positive alternative action for each one.

6. Some older students offer to drive you to a party where alcohol will be served.

_____

7. At your new school, your classmate asks if you want to go off campus to have lunch and smoke cigarettes.

_____

Activity 15

Applying Health Skills

Recognizing the Signs of a Problem

People can experience a variety of anxiety disorders, personality disorders, and mood disorders. Each of the various disorders of each type has recognizable symptoms. Read the descriptions of each of the following situations. Write the letter of the disorder that best matches the situation described.

_____ 1. Jennifer never goes into crowded places. If she stumbles into a crowd, her heart begins pounding wildly, she starts sweating and trembling, she finds herself short of breath, and she feels nauseated.

_____ 2. George takes medications to prevent the hallucinations that used to trouble him. Before starting on the drugs, he often heard or saw things that were not really there.

_____ 3. Mary has been very restless and tired lately. She has difficulty concentrating, is often irritable, and has had problems sleeping at night. Her muscles also seem to be very tense most of the time.

| a. general anxiety disorder |
| b. panic disorder |
| c. phobia |
| d. obsessive-compulsive disorder |
| e. post-traumatic stress disorder |
| f. schizophrenia |
| g. clinical depression |
| h. bipolar disorder |

_____ 4. Roseanne experiences extreme mood swings. Sometimes she feels elated and full of energy. Her mood can change dramatically, however, and she will feel depressed, tired, and desolate.

_____ 5. Since being injured in a car crash, Brad has felt very depressed, tired, and withdrawn. He seems to have no energy and does not feel like being around his friends.

_____ 6. Mark has felt depressed for weeks. His friends are concerned because he has lost interest in everything and does not seem to find enjoyment in anything that he used to like to do.

_____ 7. Jane has an irrational fear of spiders. If she sees one, she sometimes becomes frozen with fear.

_____ 8. Tina washes her hands dozens of times a day, even when she has no reason to do so. She also spends hours each day arranging her clothes and other possessions, and she checks over and over again to make sure that she has locked the doors of her house.

Activity 16

Applying Health Skills

Getting Help, Feeling Better

Read the descriptions below of some situations teens can find themselves in. On the lines following each description, state what the person can do to get help.

Situation 1

José's parents have been arguing a lot lately. He is very upset and worried that they may be thinking about getting divorced.

1. What can José do?

_____

_____

Situation 2

Paula has been getting bad grades in school. Her parents have told her that she will have to quit the soccer team and the nature club until her grades improve.

2. What can Paula do?

_____

_____

Situation 3

Some of Reggie's friends have begun using drugs. Their behavior makes Reggie very uncomfortable.

3. What can Reggie do?

_____

_____

Situation 4

Joan's friend Teresa has been feeling terrible. Her boyfriend broke up with her. Her grades are slipping. She has not slept well in weeks. She has been keeping to herself a lot lately.

4. What can Joan do?

_____

_____

Activity 17

Applying Health Skills

Dealing with Grief

Someday you may be faced with the opportunity to help someone deal with grief. Fill in the chart below to use as a guide.

Who Died	Helpful Responses
Friend's dog is killed by a car	
Friend's grandparent dies of old age	
Friend's parent dies after a long illness	

People who experience the death of a loved one may go through various stages of grief, including shock, anger, yearning, depression, and moving on. Read the descriptions below and identify the stage of grief that each individual is experiencing.

_____ 1. Laura's grandfather died several months ago. He used to come over to her house for dinner once a week. Laura is beginning to come to terms with the fact that he will not be coming to her house anymore.

_____ 2. The recent death of his wife has left Matthew feeling numb and empty inside. He wonders how he will be able to live without her.

_____ 3. Robert and Isabel feel a great ache over the death of their father. Their lives feel terribly empty, and every day they wish that he would somehow come back to them.

_____ 4. The deep pain Barbara felt when her husband died has lessened. Although she will never forget him, she has begun to look ahead and plan for the future.

_____ 5. Ted feels very angry over the death of his mother, and he blames her for leaving him.

Chapter **4** Health Inventory

Rate Your Mental and Emotional Health

Read the statements below. In the space at the left, write *yes* if the statement describes you, or *no* if it does not describe you.

_____ 1. I feel okay about expressing my feelings.

_____ 2. I enjoy my own company.

_____ 3. I can give and accept compliments.

_____ 4. I can say no to people without feeling guilty.

_____ 5. I am satisfied with my effort if I have done my best.

_____ 6. I know my limits as well as my abilities.

_____ 7. I can cope with disappointment.

_____ 8. I continue to participate in an activity even if I do not always get my way.

_____ 9. I can laugh at myself.

_____ 10. I like who I am.

_____ 11. I can ask for help when I need it.

_____ 12. I am interested in other people.

_____ 13. I set realistic goals for myself.

_____ 14. I see challenges as opportunities for growth.

_____ 15. I face my problems rather than avoid them.

Score yourself:

How many *yes* answers did you have? Write that number here.

12–15: You have excellent mental and emotional health.

8–11: Your mental and emotional health is good.

5–7: Your mental and emotional health is fair, but it could be better.

Fewer than 5: Reread Chapter 4 carefully to see what changes you can make to improve your mental and emotional health.

Chapter 5 Study Guide

STUDY TIPS

✔ Read the chapter objectives.

✔ Look up any unfamiliar words.

✔ Read the questions below before you read the chapter.

As you read the chapter, answer the following questions. Later you can use this guide to review the information in the chapter.

Lesson 1

1. Define *character*, and explain its importance to social health.

_____

_____

2. Identify three primary traits of good character.

_____

3. Name three ways to improve your relationships.

_____

_____

Lesson 2

4. Explain the function and importance of families.

_____

_____

5. List three common changes and challenges that families may face.

_____

_____

6. Explain how families contribute to a person's health triangle.

_____

_____

_____

_____

_____

7. Identify three recent trends affecting family structure.

_____

_____

8. Name three ways to help strengthen your family.

_____

_____

_____

Lesson 3

9. Identify three factors that can help a marriage succeed.

_____

_____

_____

10. Describe the role of parenting.

_____

_____

11. Name three qualities of good parenting.

_____

_____

_____

_____

_____

12. List two consequences of teen parenting.

_____

_____

_____

Activity 18 Applying Health Skills

Displaying Good Character

People with good character demonstrate trustworthiness, respect, responsibility, fairness, caring, and citizenship. For each situation below, identify the good character trait or traits that the individual demonstrates.

Situation 1
Jared has been more considerate to his parents lately. Instead of talking back to them and acting disrespectful, he is being more polite, controlling his temper, and letting them know where he is and what he's doing when he's not at home.

Character trait(s): _____

Situation 2
When Heather's soccer coach asked her to take turns being captain with Venita, Heather happily agreed. Venita is shy, and Heather thinks that being captain will be good for Venita's self-esteem.

Character trait(s): _____

Situation 3
Concerned about the environment, Bonnie talked to her principal about starting a recycling program at the school. The principal agreed and suggested that Bonnie organize the program because he knew he could rely on her.

Character trait(s): _____

Situation 4
Mario heard others making fun of the new student in his class, who speaks with a foreign accent. Mario told them that they should not make fun of people just because they are different. He then went over to talk to the boy and be friendly to him.

Character trait(s): _____

Applying Health Skills

Family Counseling Hot Line

Assume that you are a counselor answering telephone calls to a crisis hot line. On the lines beneath each problem, write the advice you would give.

Caller 1

"I'm 13 years old, and my parents still want to make all my decisions for me. They won't even allow me to choose my own clothes, much less my friends. What can I do to show them that I'm more grown-up than they think?"

My advice would be:

_____

_____

_____

Caller 2

"I know my older sister has started drinking, not just now and then, but a lot. Her friends all drink, and right now she'd do anything to make them like her. She's missing work a lot and getting really low grades. I'd like to help, but I don't know what to do."

My advice would be:

_____

_____

_____

Caller 3

"Dad's always tired and busy because he works long hours. I never get to spend any time with him. I wish we could talk about things the way we used to. What should I do?"

My advice would be:

_____

_____

_____

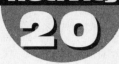

Activity 20   Applying Health Skills

Marriage and Parenthood

Sometimes young people have unrealistic ideas about marriage and parenthood. Imagine how you would respond to the following statements. Write a response on the lines below to show that you understand the responsibilities of marriage and parenthood.

1. "Getting married young will give us the opportunity to grow up together."

_____

_____

2. "We love each other. That's all we need to have a good marriage."

_____

_____

3. "What's the big deal about taking care of a baby? I've taken care of my little brother and sister lots of times."

_____

_____

4. "My girlfriend and I are having a baby. We plan to get married and find an apartment where we can be on our own. Then we can do whatever we want."

_____

_____

5. "My boyfriend will quit school and work full-time. Then we'll be able to afford to bring up our baby."

_____

_____

Chapter 5 Health Inventory

Building Character

Read the statements below. In the space at the left, put a check next to each statement that applies to you.

_____ 1. I am a loyal and reliable person.

_____ 2. I always play by the rules.

_____ 3. I work to make my community a better place.

_____ 4. I am always polite and well-mannered.

_____ 5. I treat property with care.

_____ 6. Before acting on a thought or feeling, I think of the consequences of my actions.

_____ 7. I try to help others who are in need.

_____ 8. I practice good sportsmanship.

_____ 9. I always let my parents know where I am and what I'm doing.

_____ 10. I obey the rules in my school.

_____ 11. I am tolerant of other people's differences.

_____ 12. I always try to do my best in whatever I undertake.

_____ 13. I care about the feelings of others.

_____ 14. I accept responsibility for my mistakes or for things I do that are wrong.

_____ 15. I take turns and share with other people.

Score yourself:

Write the number of checks here.

11–15: You display excellent character.

6–10: Your character is good but could use improvement.

Fewer than 6: You need to work harder to develop good character.

Chapter Study Guide

STUDY TIPS
✔ Read the chapter objectives.
✔ Look up any unfamiliar words.
✔ Read the questions below before you read the chapter.

As you read the chapter, answer the following questions. Later you can use this guide to review the information in the chapter.

Lesson 1

1. Explain how friendship changes from childhood to the teen years.

_____

_____

2. Identify four qualities of a good friendship.

_____

_____

3. List three tips for making new friends.

_____

_____

4. Define *clique*, and explain how cliques can have a positive influence.

_____

_____

_____

Lesson 2

5. Contrast positive and negative peer pressure.

_____

_____

_____

_____

6. Describe three ways to deal with negative peer pressure.

_____

_____

_____

_____

7. List the four steps of effective refusal skills.

_____

_____

_____

_____

Lesson 3

8. Define *limits*, and explain why they are important.

_____

_____

_____

_____

9. Identify three ways to show affection without being sexually active.

_____

_____

_____

_____

10. List four rewards of sexual abstinence.

_____

_____

_____

_____

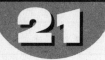

Activity 21

Use with Chapter 6, Lesson 1.

Applying Health Skills

Qualities of Good Friends

Although friends may be different from each other, good friendships share similar qualities.

Look at the qualities of friendship listed at the right. Read each quote. In the space after each quote, write the letter of the quality the quote expresses.

1. "I'm sorry about your cat. I know how I felt when my dog was sick."

_____

2. "I don't agree with what you're saying, but I understand your position."

_____

3. "I know how important it is to complete my part of the assignment. I'll be sure to have it done on time."

_____

4. "I'm so excited about being accepted into the exchange program, but I'm not telling anyone but you until I'm sure I can go!"

_____

5. "How are you feeling?"

_____

a.	caring
b.	empathy
c.	reliability
d.	respect
e.	trust

Activity 22 — Applying Health Skills

Some Good Advice

What advice would you give to the teens in the situations described below? Write your answers on the lines provided.

Situation 1
Someone offers Lonny a cigarette, but he knows that smoking is unhealthful.

_____

_____

Situation 2
Some of Carla's friends have started dating and have told her that they think she should, too. Carla does not feel ready to date. She is sure that there are other teens at school who feel the way she does.

_____

_____

Situation 3
Wesley has begun to wonder whether to remain friends with Ted, who has started doing things Wesley does not approve of. Sometimes Ted asks Wesley to join him.

_____

_____

Situation 4
Some of Nick's friends have suggested that they all crash a neighborhood party.

_____

_____

Situation 5
Michelle is being pressured by some of her friends to drink alcohol.

_____

_____

Activity 23   Applying Health Skills

How Far Should I Go?

Setting limits protects individuals from risky or unhealthful behaviors. This can be especially important in dealing with sexual activity. Answer the questions below concerning the ways teens can set limits on sexual behaviors and the benefits of doing so.

Showing Affection

List four ways that a person can show affection without being sexually active.

_____

_____

_____

Supporting Abstinence

Identify four ways to be a role model for friends who are seeking ways to promote abstinence from sexual activity before marriage.

_____

_____

_____

_____

Avoiding Consequences

Name three possible consequences of sexual activity.

_____

Rewards of Abstinence

List rewards of sexual abstinence.

_____

_____

_____

Chapter 6 Health Inventory

Rate Your Relationships with Your Friends and Peers

Rate yourself as a friend by circling *yes* or *no* for each item below.

yes	no	**1.** My friends and I respect each other's opinions.
yes	no	**2.** My friends and I can trust each other.
yes	no	**3.** I try to have a positive influence on my friends and peers.
yes	no	**4.** I am able to make new friends.
yes	no	**5.** I try to plan fun, safe activities with my friends.
yes	no	**6.** My friends and I can depend on each other.
yes	no	**7.** My friends and I care about each other.
yes	no	**8.** I am able to use refusal skills to deal with negative peer pressure.
yes	no	**9.** My friends and I can count on each other to keep our promises.
yes	no	**10.** I do not pressure people to do things that they believe are wrong.
yes	no	**11.** I avoid risky dating situations.
yes	no	**12.** I express affection in healthy ways.
yes	no	**13.** My friends have a positive influence on me.
yes	no	**14.** My friends and I are empathetic with each other.
yes	no	**15.** My friends know that I care what happens to them.

Score yourself:

How many *yes* answers did you circle? Write that number here.

11–15: You deserve top honors for your good friend and peer relationships.

6–10: You have average relationships with your friends and peers.

Fewer than 6: Changing some of your actions will allow you to have more valuable relationships with your friends and peers.

Chapter 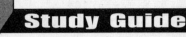 7 Study Guide

As you read the chapter, answer the following questions. Later you can use this guide to review the information in the chapter.

Lesson 1

1. Define *conflict*.

_____

2. What are the three major reasons for conflict?

_____

3. Name three factors that can cause minor conflicts to escalate into major disputes.

_____

Lesson 2

4. What are the principles of conflict resolution?

_____

_____

5. Name four skills you can use if you are involved in a conflict.

_____

_____

6. Define *mediation*, and identify two qualities and skills of an effective mediator.

_____

_____

7. What are the six steps in the mediation process?

_____

_____

_____

_____

8. What is *peer mediation?*

_____

Lesson 3

9. Define *violence*, and identify two factors that are thought to contribute to high levels of violence in society.

_____

_____

_____

10. Identify three typical gang activities.

_____

_____

11. List three ways to protect yourself from violence.

_____

_____

Lesson 4

12. Define *abuse*, and identify four basic forms of abuse.

_____

_____

13. Define *sexual harassment.*

_____

_____

14. Identify four resources for getting help for abuse.

_____

Activity 24 · Applying Health Skills

Identifying Conflicts

Read about the conflicts described below. For each one, write the causes of the conflict and the factors that could cause it to get out of hand. Then suggest how each conflict might be resolved or managed.

What Causes Conflicts	Why Conflicts Get Out of Hand
resources	anger
values	bullying and teasing
emotional needs	group pressure

Conflict 1

Roberto and Carlos both want to use the family computer. Roberto wants to play a game, but Carlos wants to search the Internet for free software. Roberto teases Carlos and calls him a computer geek. Carlos gets angry and threatens to dump Roberto's games from the computer.

Cause(s): _____ Escalating Factor(s): _____

Suggested Resolution(s): _____

_____

Conflict 2

Brian loves rap music, but his older brother thinks that it's just noise. One morning Brian's brother turns down the volume on Brian's radio so hard that he breaks the knob. All day at school Brian thinks about what his brother did. That night they quarrel over what to watch on television.

Cause(s): _____ Escalating Factor(s): _____

Suggested Resolution(s): _____

_____

Conflict 3

Selena joins Betty and her friends at a school cafeteria table. They make fun of the food Selena's mother packed in her lunch. Selena responds by saying that Betty's lunch will make her fat. Betty, upset, leads her friends to another table. Selena is left alone, feeling humiliated and thinking about what Betty has done.

Cause(s): _____ Escalating Factor(s): _____

Suggested Resolution(s): _____

_____

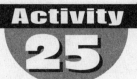

Applying Health Skills

Resolving Conflicts

You can use the peer mediation process to resolve conflicts. Below are mixed-up quotes from students in conflict about the use of a neighborhood basketball court. Place the letter by each quote in the correct box to show how the steps of the peer mediation process were followed and how the conflict was resolved.

Quotes

a. "Maybe we could take turns using the court on different days, or we could schedule certain hours for each group every afternoon and on weekends."

b. "All right, I've heard your group's side of the story. Now let me hear how the other guys see it."

c. "What do you guys think you're doing? We use this basketball court. You guys are new to the neighborhood, so you'll have to find someplace else to play."

d. "As long as we keep to the schedule, and each group gets equal time on the court, I guess it's okay with us."

e. "Wait a minute. Let's talk this out with a peer mediator."

f. "Sorry we got in your face about this. We should have talked it out first before getting angry about it."

g. "Look, we've been playing on this court since last year. They just moved into the neighborhood. We have more of a right to play here than they do."

The Peer Mediation Process

Conflict!	
Parties agree to negotiate.	
Mediator listens to each point of view.	
Parties clarify their wants and needs.	
They brainstorm possible solutions.	
They evaluate their solutions.	
Conflict is resolved.	

Activity 26 Applying Health Skills

On Guard Against Violence

Read each of the situations below, and indicate whether it poses a *risk* for violence or represents a *precaution* against violence. The first two have been done for you.

_____risk_____ 1. Mark and his two best friends use illegal drugs regularly.

__precaution__ 2. Bonnie always locks the doors and windows when she's home alone.

_____ 3. When Carlos walks alone in the city, he always stands tall and tries to walk with an air of confidence.

_____ 4. After work each night, Freddi usually walks home alone along several poorly lit streets in a deserted part of town.

_____ 5. Rhonda's boyfriend is a member of a gang, and she often hangs out with him and the other gang members.

_____ 6. Martin's school adopted a zero tolerance policy for weapons and drugs.

_____ 7. Caitlyn likes to drink when she goes out on dates, even when she's with boys she doesn't know very well.

_____ 8. When someone calls Wendy's house and asks for her parents while she's home alone, she says that her parents are busy right now and will call the person back later.

_____ 9. Although his parents have warned him not to hitchhike, Darryl has done it a number of times.

_____ 10. Since he was beaten up by classmates last year, Nelson now carries a knife with him to school.

_____ 11. Ana always carries enough cash with her on dates so that she can call a cab to get home if necessary.

_____ 12. The town in which Kendra lives installed lighting in all parks and playgrounds last year.

_____ 13. Terrell loves chatting on the Internet and doesn't mind giving out personal information about himself.

_____ 14. Kimberly sometimes goes to secluded areas with her dates.

Activity 27 Applying Health Skills

The Facts About Abuse

In each blank, write the letter of the term that will best complete the sentence.

1. _____ is the legal term for beating, hitting, or kicking another person.

2. _____ is uninvited and unwelcome sexual conduct directed at another person that may include words, touching, jokes, looks, or gestures with sexual meaning.

3. All conversations on _____ are kept confidential.

4. Constant teasing, bullying, and threats of physical violence are forms of _____.

5. A child deprived of love and encouragement, nourishing food, clothing, adequate housing, education, safety, and medical care suffers from _____.

6. Abuse is _____ the victim's fault.

7. _____ is physical, emotional, or mental mistreatment of one person by another.

8. Family members who are in danger of being abused can often stay in _____ while they get help putting their lives in order.

9. _____ includes hitting, slapping, kicking, pushing, shoving, punching, and choking.

10. _____ occurs when one person is forced to participate in a sexual act against his or her will.

11. One key to stopping all forms of abuse is to break the _____.

a. emotional abuse
b. neglect
c. battery
d. abuse
e. never
f. physical abuse
g. sexual harassment
h. sexual abuse
i. cycle of abuse
j. shelters
k. crisis hot lines

Chapter 7 Health Inventory

Resolving Conflicts and Preventing Violence

Read the statements below. In the space at the left, write *yes* if the statement describes you, or *no* if it does not describe you.

_____ 1. I take actions to manage my anger when I feel it.

_____ 2. I am able to share resources and show respect for other people's needs.

_____ 3. I understand that the best solution to a conflict is one in which both sides win.

_____ 4. I take a time out when I am involved in a conflict.

_____ 5. I can communicate my feelings calmly and reasonably in a conflict.

_____ 6. I respect the values held by other people.

_____ 7. When I am involved in a conflict, I listen actively and make sure I understand what the other person has said.

_____ 8. I recognize that everyone shares the emotional need to feel worthwhile.

_____ 9. I always respond to bullies by walking away from the situation.

_____ 10. I take precautions at home and outdoors to protect myself from violence.

_____ 11. I know that seeking help can help to break the cycle of abuse.

_____ 12. I know that alcohol and other drugs can contribute to violence.

_____ 13. I know that no one, no matter what, deserves to be treated abusively.

_____ 14. I realize that sexual harassment is a serious issue.

_____ 15. I am aware of places where a victim of abuse can go for help.

Score yourself:

Write the number of *yes* answers here.

12–15: You are well informed about conflict resolution and violence prevention.

8–11: You need to learn more about conflict and violence.

Fewer than 8: You have some work to do to understand conflict and develop ways to avoid violence.

Chapter 8 Study Guide

STUDY TIPS

✔ Read the chapter objectives.

✔ Look up any unfamiliar words.

✔ Read the questions below before you read the chapter.

As you read the chapter, answer the following questions. Later you can use this guide to review the information in the chapter.

Lesson 1

1. What are two reasons to make nutritious food choices?

_____

2. List three important roles of nutrients.

_____

_____

3. Name four factors that influence your food choices.

_____

_____

4. Identify three elements that affect the amounts of nutrients a person needs.

_____

Lesson 2

5. List the six types of nutrients, and give one food source of each.

_____

_____

_____

_____

6. Define *fiber*, and explain how it helps the digestive system.

_____

_____

7. Identify the two types of cholesterol in the blood.

_____

_____

Lesson 3

8. Describe the three main points of the Dietary Guidelines.

_____

_____

_____

_____

9. List the food groups in MyPyramid.

_____

_____

10. List four types of information provided on all food labels.

_____

Lesson 4

11. Explain why breakfast is the most important meal of the day, and tell how eating breakfast can help teens.

_____

_____

12. Explain the importance of eating regular meals.

_____

_____

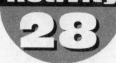

Applying Health Skills

Choices of Food

A variety of factors influence what people eat. Among these are family and friends, cultural background, food availability, time and money resources, advertising, knowledge of nutrition, and personal preferences. Read the following situations. Identify which factor or factors might have influenced the person's food choices.

Situation 1
Margot's father is from Italy. Tonight Margot is serving an antipasto salad, lasagna, and chicken cacciatore.

_____

Situation 2
While walking back to his dormitory after classes at the university, Mark stopped at a little shop and bought a small container of orange juice and a box of raisins as a snack.

_____

Situation 3
Since Annette lost her job, she has been serving lots of pasta, beans, and vegetables to her children.

_____

Situation 4
Tyler didn't have much time for lunch. The bagel store across the street from his work was out of poppy seed bagels, so he got a sesame seed bagel instead.

_____

Situation 5
Janine, a school nurse, tries to make sure that her children always eat nutritious foods.

_____

Situation 6
Marcia purchases food based on the coupons she gets in the newspaper. She also likes to try new food that she has read about in magazines.

_____

Activity 29

Applying Health Skills

Vitamins and Minerals

Vitamins and minerals are substances the body needs to function properly. Look at the chart below, and answer the questions that follow.

Nutrient	What It Does	Where to Get It
Vitamin A	aids growth, skin, vision	dark green leafy vegetables, deep yellow-orange fruits and vegetables, eggs, liver
B vitamins	promotes healthy nervous system, helps produce energy	poultry, eggs, meat, fish, whole-grain breads and cereals
Vitamin C	promotes healthy teeth, gums, and bones; helps heal wounds and fight infection	citrus fruits, tomatoes, cabbage, broccoli
Vitamin D	promotes strong bones and teeth	fortified milk, fatty fish, egg yolks, liver
Calcium	aids strong teeth and bones	dairy products, spinach, sardines
Iron	needed for hemoglobin in red blood cells	red meat, poultry, dry beans, nuts, eggs, dried fruits, dark green vegetables
Potassium	regulates fluid balance in tissues; promotes proper nerve function	bananas, oranges, dry beans and peas, dried fruits

1. Which nutrients do you need for strong, healthy teeth? _____

2. Why is iron important? _____

3. Which vitamin is contained in fortified milk? _____

4. Which two nutrients do green vegetables provide? _____

5. Which healthy substances are in a banana split? _____

6. Which nutrients help produce energy? _____

Activity 30

Applying Health Skills

Knowing What You Eat

All packaged foods have labels headed "Nutrition Facts" that provide valuable information for making healthful food choices. Look at the food label shown here and answer the questions that follow.

1. How many calories are in each serving of this cereal?

   _____

2. What is a normal serving size?

   _____

3. How many grams of total fat does one serving contain? What percentage of the total daily fat allowance does this provide?

   _____

4. How many grams of dietary fiber are found in one serving of the cereal? What percent daily value of total dietary fiber does this provide?

   _____

5. What vitamins and minerals are found in this food product?

   _____

6. Approximately how many calories would you consume if you ate the whole box of cereal?

   _____

7. Would this be good for a person who has to restrict the intake of sodium? Why?

   _____

8. Which ingredients listed are not in the Grains Group?

   _____

Crunchy Oats
Nutrition Facts
Serving Size ½ Cup (50 g)
Servings Per Container about 8

Amount per serving	
Calories	240
Calories from Fat	80

	% **Daily Value***
Total Fat 9.5g	14%
Saturated Fat 1g	5%
Cholesterol 0mg	0%
Sodium 0mg	0%
Total Carbohydrate 35g	11%
Dietary Fiber 8g	22%
Sugars 8g	
Protein 7g	

Vitamin A	<3%
Vitamin C	<2%
Calcium	4%
Iron	7%

*Percent Daily Values are based on a 2,000 calorie diet. Your daily values may be higher or lower depending on your calorie needs.

INGREDIENTS: OATS, GRAPE CONCENTRATE, RICE CRISP (RICE FLOUR, MALT, RICE BRAN), RAISINS, ALMONDS, PINE NUTS, SESAME SEEDS, SAFFLOWER OIL, OAT SYRUP, NATURAL VANILLA FLAVOR, NATURAL VITAMIN E (TO PRESERVE FRESHNESS).

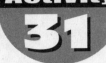

Activity 31

Applying Health Skills

Menu Planning

The key to a balanced eating plan is advance planning. Prepare a menu plan for the next three days by completing the chart below. Be sure to include the five main food groups in the menus for each day.

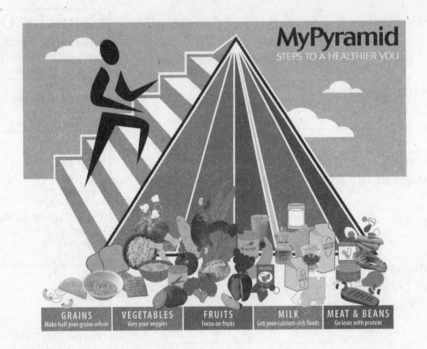

Menu Plan			
	Day 1	Day 2	Day 3
Breakfast			
Lunch			
Snack			
Dinner			

Chapter 8 Health Inventory

How Healthy Are Your Food Habits?

Read each statement below. Decide how it describes your food behavior. Write *always*, *sometimes*, or *never* in the space at the left of each statement.

_____ 1. I pay attention to the nutrients in foods.

_____ 2. I try to eat plenty of calcium-rich foods.

_____ 3. I eat breakfast every day.

_____ 4. I choose healthful, low-fat snacks.

_____ 5. I eat plenty of fruits and vegetables.

_____ 6. I limit my intake of caffeine.

_____ 7. I read the labels on food packages.

_____ 8. I balance my food intake with physical activity.

_____ 9. I eat mostly lean meats.

_____ 10. I help my family plan nutritious meals.

_____ 11. I use low-fat or nonfat milk with cereal.

_____ 12. I eat foods that are rich in fiber.

_____ 13. I limit my intake of foods that are high in fat or sugar.

_____ 14. I try not to eat on the run.

_____ 15. I eat when I'm hungry.

Score yourself:

Give yourself 3 points for each *always* answer, 1 point for each *sometimes*, and 0 for each *never*. Write your score here.

36–45: Very good

26–35: Good

16–25: Room for improvement

Fewer than 16: Take a close look at your food patterns, and see what changes you can make.

Chapter 9 Study Guide

STUDY TIPS

✔ Read the chapter objectives.

✔ Look up any unfamiliar words.

✔ Read the questions below before you read the chapter.

As you read the chapter, answer the following questions. Later you can use this guide to review the information in the chapter.

Lesson 1

1. Explain the difference between the terms *physical activity*, *exercise*, and *physical fitness*.

_____

_____

_____

2. Identify three social benefits of physical activity.

_____

_____

3. Name the two types of exercise, and give two examples of each.

_____

Lesson 2

4. Name the four major elements of physical fitness.

_____

5. List two types of cardiovascular exercise that can help build heart and lung endurance.

_____

6. Define *flexibility*.

_____

7. Explain the difference between muscle strength and muscle endurance.

_____

_____

_____

Lesson 3

8. Name three things you can do to be active every day.

_____

_____

_____

9. List the three stages of exercise workouts.

_____

10. Identify and describe four guidelines for the work out stage of an exercise program.

_____

_____

_____

_____

Lesson 4

11. List two advantages of individual sports.

_____

_____

12. List two advantages of team sports.

_____

_____

_____

13. Identify three tips for practicing safe behavior and preventing sports-related injuries.

_____

_____

_____

Activity 32

Applying Health Skills

Fitness Facts and Myths

Some of the statements below are facts; others are not. Classify each by writing *fact* or *myth* in the space at the left. On the lines that follow the statements, correct the ones you have identified as myths.

_____ 1. Physical fitness improves your ability to meet the physical demands of daily life.

_____

_____ 2. Regular exercise alone will allow you to be fit.

_____

_____ 3. Only people who are physically fit should participate in regular physical activity.

_____

_____ 4. Physical activity increases a person's self-confidence and self-esteem.

_____

_____ 5. Being physically active can strengthen your heart and lungs.

_____

_____ 6. Aerobic exercise alone will help you achieve optimum fitness.

_____

_____ 7. For an exercise to be effective, it should be done three to five times a week.

_____

_____ 8. Physical activity helps reduce stress.

_____

_____ 9. Modern technology has replaced many physical activities that were once part of daily life.

_____

_____ 10. Exercise enables a person to enjoy life more.

_____

Activity 33 — Applying Health Skills

Elements of Fitness

Read the physical fitness test results for the people below. Rate each person's physical fitness as *acceptable* or *needs improvement*. Also indicate what the person's target pulse rate during exercise should be.

1. Ed is 13 years old. In the test for heart and lung endurance, he walked 2.3 miles in 30 minutes. For upper body strength and endurance, he kept his chin above the bar for 16 seconds. In the test for abdominal strength and endurance, he did 38 curl-ups. He was able to reach 3 inches in the flexibility test.

   Rating: _____

   Target Pulse Rate: _____

2. Jackie is 15 years old. In the test for heart and lung endurance, she walked 1 mile in 30 minutes. For upper body strength and endurance, she kept her chin above the bar for 5 seconds. In the test for abdominal strength and endurance, she did 15 curl-ups. She could not reach her toes in the flexibility test.

   Rating: _____

   Target Pulse Rate: _____

3. Margo is 12 years old. In the test for heart and lung endurance, she jogged 1.8 miles in 20 minutes. For upper body strength and endurance, she kept her chin above the bar for 13 seconds. In the test for abdominal strength and endurance, she did 33 curl-ups. She reached 3 inches in the flexibility test.

   Rating: _____

   Target Pulse Rate: _____

4. Colin is 14 years old. In the test for heart and lung endurance, he jogged 1.3 miles in 20 minutes. For upper body strength and endurance, he kept his chin above the bar for 8 seconds. In the test for abdominal strength and endurance, he did 24 curl-ups. He was able to just touch his toes in the flexibility test.

   Rating: _____

   Target Pulse Rate: _____

Activity 34

Use with Chapter 9, Lesson 3.

Applying Health Skills

Keeping Fit

Physical activity and exercise can help you both manage weight and control blood pressure and blood sugar. As important as exercise is, it is equally important to know how much and what kind of exercise to do. Walking and bicycle riding are both popular forms of exercise. The following charts show suggestions for a walking and a bicycling program.

Read the charts and answer the questions below.

Walking Program

Steps	Plan	Time
Step 1	Walk at an easy pace	15 minutes
Step 2	Walk faster, covering 1.5 miles	30 minutes
Step 3	Walk as in step 2, covering 2 miles	40 minutes
Step 4	Walk a bit faster, covering 3 miles	40 minutes

Bicycling Program

Steps	Plan	Time
Step 1	Pedal at an easy pace	5 to 10 minutes
Step 2	Bicycle faster, covering 3 miles	25 minutes
Step 3	Bicycle a bit faster, covering 4 miles	25 minutes
Step 4	Bicycle a bit faster, covering 5 miles	25 minutes

1. Mrs. Horowitz tries to ride her bicycle 3 times a week. It takes her about 5 minutes to cover each mile. What step is she up to?

_____

2. Susan is now used to her bike. She had spent a week or so going along at easy speeds for about 10 minutes a day, building up her conditioning. What should she do now?

_____

3. Mr. Ramsey spent 3 weeks at step 2 in the walking program. Now he is at step 3 and is just barely able to cover 2 miles in 40 minutes. What do you suggest he do?

_____

Activity 35

Applying Health Skills

Individual and Team Sports

Use your knowledge of individual and team sports to complete the following chart. In the first column, list ten individual or team sports that interest you. Then, in each appropriate column, note whether each sport you listed is a team or individual sport, the equipment needed to participate (if any), and why the sport interests you.

Sport	Individual/ Team Sport?	Equipment Needed?	Why Am I Interested in This Sport?

Chapter 9 Health Inventory

How Good Are Your Fitness Habits?

Read each statement below. Decide how it describes your fitness habits. Write *always*, *sometimes*, or *never* in the space at the left of each statement.

_____ 1. I walk or ride my bike to school.

_____ 2. I take the stairs rather than an elevator or escalator if I can.

_____ 3. When my friends are deciding what to do for fun, I suggest an active game or sport such as swimming, basketball, or hiking.

_____ 4. I participate in an active game, sport, or work activity every day.

_____ 5. I rest for a while after a vigorous game or activity.

_____ 6. I eat a balanced, nutritious diet.

_____ 7. I warm up before every exercise session.

_____ 8. I cool down after each exercise session.

_____ 9. I exercise three to five times every week.

_____ 10. I choose safe places, such as soft, even surfaces rather than a street, to exercise.

_____ 11. I choose a safe time to exercise.

_____ 12. I drink plenty of fluids during exercise.

_____ 13. I pay attention to signals from my body, such as pain, when I exercise.

_____ 14. I wear shoes and equipment that fit correctly and are appropriate for the activity.

_____ 15. When I snack, I choose nutritious foods, such as fruit.

Score yourself:

Give yourself 3 points for each *always* answer, 1 point for each *sometimes* answer, and 0 for each *never*. Write your score here.

36–45: Your fitness habits are very good.

26–35: You have good fitness habits.

16–25: You have room for improvement.

Fewer than 16: Review your fitness habits, and plan to achieve some fitness goals!

Chapter 10 Study Guide

STUDY TIPS

✔ Read the chapter objectives.

✔ Look up any unfamiliar words.

✔ Read the questions below before you read the chapter.

   As you read the chapter, answer the following questions. Later you can use this guide to review the information in the chapter.

Lesson 1

1. Define *body image*, and explain how it can affect self-image.

_____

_____

2. Identify three factors that influence a person's appropriate weight.

_____

_____

3. Define *Body Mass Index (BMI)*, and explain its purpose.

_____

_____

4. List two harmful effects of being overweight.

_____

_____

_____

5. Identify two harmful effects of being underweight.

_____

_____

6. Explain the relationship between calories and weight gain or loss.

_____

_____

Lesson 2

7. Identify two factors that can lead to eating disorders.

_____

_____

_____

8. Name three psychological factors that can trigger eating disorders.

_____

_____

_____

9. Define *anorexia nervosa*, and describe how it can damage the body.

_____

_____

_____

10. Define *bulimia*, and describe how it can damage the body.

_____

_____

_____

_____

11. Define *binge eating disorder*, and describe how this disorder can damage the body.

_____

_____

_____

_____

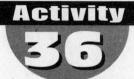

Activity 36

Applying Health Skills

Losing Weight

Two eating plans for losing weight are described below. Read the descriptions, and answer the questions that follow each description.

Roger's Eating Plan

Roger wants to lose a few pounds. He has read about an all-protein diet guaranteed to take off 14 pounds in 14 days. Roger has cottage cheese for breakfast, a cheeseburger for lunch, and a steak for dinner. As the diet instructed, he drinks eight glasses of water each day. Roger is losing weight, but he is very grumpy and does not seem to have much energy.

1. What is wrong with Roger's eating plan?

_____

_____

2. How should Roger change his eating plan?

_____

_____

Claudia's Eating Plan

Claudia wants to lose 5 pounds before the junior prom. She has decided to have a boiled egg, grapefruit juice, and toast for breakfast. For lunch she will eat a piece of baked chicken left over from last night's dinner with carrot and celery sticks. Claudia's after-school snack will be a glass of low-fat milk and an apple. At dinner she will eat whatever is prepared for the family, but she will not have butter or sour cream on her potato, and she will have fruit instead of layer cake for dessert.

3. Explain why Claudia's eating plan is likely to be successful.

_____

_____

4. Explain why Claudia's eating plan is healthful.

_____

_____

Activity 37

Use with Chapter 10, Lesson 2.

Applying Health Skills

Eating Disorders

Write a short paragraph about anorexia nervosa, describing the
signs and dangers of the disorder.

_____

_____

_____

_____

_____

Write a short paragraph about bulimia, describing the signs and
dangers of the disorder.

_____

_____

_____

_____

_____

Write a short paragraph about binge eating disorder, describing
its signs and dangers.

_____

_____

_____

_____

_____

Chapter 10 Health Inventory

How Well Do You Manage Your Weight?

Read each statement below. In the space at the left, write *yes* if the statement describes you, or *no* if it does not describe you.

_____ 1. I feel good about my body.

_____ 2. I am an appropriate weight for my age, gender, height, and body frame.

_____ 3. I avoid eating at fast-food places.

_____ 4. I try to get regular physical activity every day.

_____ 5. I try to limit my fat intake to less than 30 percent of the total calories I eat each day.

_____ 6. I pay close attention to the nutrient value of the foods I eat.

_____ 7. I base my food choices on the Food Guide Pyramid.

_____ 8. I pay attention to portion sizes when I'm eating.

_____ 9. I drink water or fruit juice instead of a soft drink when I'm thirsty.

_____ 10. I avoid fad diets.

_____ 11. I set realistic goals for maintaining my weight.

_____ 12. I avoid using food as a way to cope with depression or stress.

_____ 13. I seek the support of family and friends when I'm feeling bad about my body or my weight.

_____ 14. I talk to my doctor if I am concerned about my weight.

_____ 15. I focus on how I feel rather than on how I look.

Score yourself:

Write the number of *yes* answers here.

12–15: Excellent

8–11: Good

Fewer than 8: You need to do a better job of managing your weight.

Chapter Study Guide

   As you read the chapter, answer the following questions. Later you can use this guide to review the information in the chapter.

Lesson 1

1. Explain the difference between _drugs_ and _medicines._

_____

_____

2. List four pieces of information that appear on prescription medicine labels.

_____

_____

_____

3. Explain what a _vaccine_ is and what it does.

_____

_____

Lesson 2

4. Explain the difference between _drug misuse_ and _drug abuse._

_____

_____

_____

5. Explain why narcotics are dangerous, and name two prescription narcotics.

_____

6. Explain the difference between *stimulants* and *depressants*.

_____

Lesson 3

7. Describe three harmful effects of using marijuana.

_____

_____

_____

8. Name two negative effects of PCP.

_____

_____

_____

9. Identify two commonly used club drugs.

_____

Lesson 4

10. List five reasons for choosing to be drug free.

_____

_____

_____

_____

_____

11. Identify three ways to help yourself live a drug-free life.

_____

_____

_____

Activity 38 — Applying Health Skills

Evaluating OTC Drugs

Some medications can be bought without prescriptions from a doctor. This sheet will help you evaluate some of these over-the-counter (OTC) drugs. To answer the questions below, visit a drugstore, examine your home medicine cabinet, or look at newspaper advertisements for over-the-counter products.

1. List four different kinds of over-the-counter medications, and give a brand name example of each kind.

Kinds of OTC Medications	Brand Name Examples
a.	
b.	
c.	
d.	

2. Choose two examples of over-the-counter products. Complete the chart below by answering the questions about the two products.

	Product 1	Product 2
a. brand name		
b. purpose		
c. directions for use		
d. typical dosage (amount used each time)		
e. cost per dose		
f. side effects and warnings		

3. What type of over-the-counter medication do you consider most helpful? Why?

4. What type of over-the-counter medication do you consider least helpful? Why?

Activity 39 — Applying Health Skills

Letter Scramble

Unscramble the capitalized words in the sentences below. Then write the words on the lines at the left. On the numbered lines at the bottom of the page, write the circled letters from the words you have unscrambled. They will form a four-word message.

_ _ ◯ _ _ _   1. Not following a doctor's directions when taking a drug is drug SIMEUS.

_ _ _ ◯ _ _ _   2. ICCONEA is an addictive stimulant drug known as coke.

_ _ _ ◯ _ _   3. Amphetamine is a drug that stimulates the central nervous MYSETS.

_ _ _ _ _ ◯ _   4. DIOCEEN is a prescription narcotic sometimes used to treat pain.

_ _ _ ◯ _   5. Abusing depressants can result in MACO.

_ _ _ _ _ ◯ _ _ _ _ _   6. One group of illegal stimulant drugs are SPANETHIMAME.

_ _ _ _ ◯ _ _ _   7. CRITOSCAN are drugs prescribed to relieve severe pain.

_ _ _ ◯ _ _ _ _ _   8. Drug DADITCNIO is a physical or psychological need for a drug.

_ _ ◯ _ _   9. KARCC is a very dangerous concentrated form of cocaine.

_ _ _ ◯ _ _ _ _ _   10. Caffeine is a LISTMUNAT.

_ _ _ ◯ _   11. GRUD abuse includes using illegal substances.

_ _ _ _ ◯ _ _ _ _ _   12. Tranquilizers are one form of TRASPENDES.

<u>1</u> <u>2</u> <u>3</u>   <u>4</u> <u>5</u>   <u>6</u> <u>7</u>   <u>8</u> <u>9</u> <u>10</u> <u>11</u> <u>12</u>

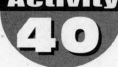

Applying Health Skills

Drug Fact Finding

Some of the statements below are true; others are not. Classify each by writing *true* or *false* on the line at the left. On the lines that follow the statements, correct the ones you have identified as false.

_____ 1. Street drugs include only illegal drugs such as heroin.

_____

_____ 2. Hallucinogens cause the body to fight off germs.

_____

_____ 3. Marijuana is stronger than hashish.

_____

_____ 4. Smoking marijuana helps people think more clearly.

_____

_____ 5. Marijuana can interfere with the way the body produces hormones.

_____

_____ 6. Marijuana does not affect a user's ability to drive a car.

_____

_____ 7. Club drugs are safe drugs.

_____

_____ 8. The effects of PCP last only several minutes.

_____

_____ 9. The use of LSD can cause terrifying thoughts and feelings.

_____

_____ 10. Nail polish remover and spray paint are legal, so inhaling their fumes cannot harm the body.

_____

_____

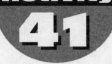

Activity
41

Applying Health Skills

Your Antidrug Campaign

Imagine that you are planning an antidrug campaign. As part of your campaign, you will design a T-shirt, a bumper sticker, a billboard, and a lapel button. Write the slogans you propose to use on the sketches below.

A.

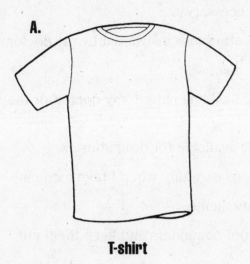

T-shirt

B.

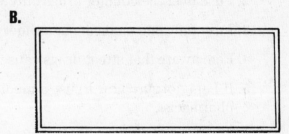

Bumper Sticker

C.

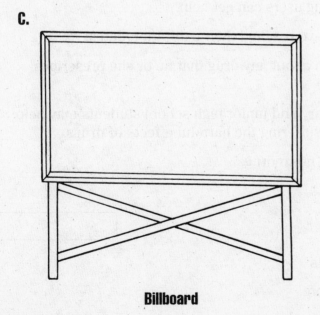

Billboard

D.

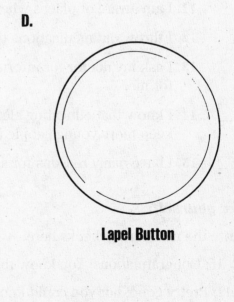

Lapel Button

Chapter **11** Health Inventory

Drug Facts, Behavior, and Attitudes

Here is a checklist about drug facts, behavior, and attitudes. In the space at the left, put a check next to each statement that describes you.

_____ **1.** I understand the differences between types of drugs.

_____ **2.** I use over-the-counter drugs only when necessary.

_____ **3.** I use only one medicine at a time, unless otherwise instructed by my doctor.

_____ **4.** I am aware that street drugs cause many deaths.

_____ **5.** If I am not sure how to use a medication, I ask my parent, my doctor, or the pharmacist.

_____ **6.** I know that there are treatment programs available for drug abusers.

_____ **7.** I read the information and follow directions carefully when I take medicine.

_____ **8.** I never share anyone else's prescription medicine.

_____ **9.** I keep medicines safely sealed in childproof containers and keep them out of the reach of children.

_____ **10.** I know that school and community activities for teens can be an alternative to drug use.

_____ **11.** I am aware of places where drug users can get help.

_____ **12.** I throw out medications that have reached their expiration dates.

_____ **13.** I ask my doctor for information about any drug that he or she prescribes for me.

_____ **14.** I know that educating elementary and junior high school students may help keep more young people from suffering the harmful effects of drugs.

_____ **15.** I have many reasons for saying no to drugs.

Score yourself:

Write the number of checks here.

12–15: Congratulations! You know the facts.

8–11: Pretty good, but you could know more.

Fewer than 8: It's time you learned the facts; they could save your life.

Chapter 12 Study Guide

As you read the chapter, answer the following questions. Later you can use this guide to review the information in the chapter.

Lesson 1

1. List the various forms of tobacco, and identify the health problems associated with each.

_____

_____

_____

2. List and define the three most harmful substances found in tobacco.

_____

_____

_____

3. What serious diseases of the respiratory, circulatory, nervous, and digestive systems can be caused by long-term tobacco use?

_____

_____

_____

4. List the ways in which smoking can affect personal appearance.

_____

_____

Lesson 2

5. Define *addiction.*

_____

6. Explain *physical* and *psychological dependence.*

_____

_____

_____

7. Identify and define the two kinds of *secondhand smoke.*

_____

_____

8. Describe the risks that tobacco products pose to unborn babies and children.

_____

_____

_____

_____

_____

Lesson 3

9. List the internal and external influences that may cause teens to start smoking.

_____

_____

_____

10. Identify three strategies that can help in resisting peer pressure to use tobacco.

_____

11. List and explain two ways to break a tobacco habit.

_____

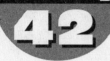

Activity 42

Applying Health Skills

Effects of Tobacco Use

No matter in what form it is used, tobacco affects every aspect of a person's life. The chemicals in tobacco can cause damage to just about every one of the body's systems. Answer the questions below concerning the specific ways in which tobacco affects the body.

Personal Appearance

List four ways in which tobacco use can affect a person's personal appearance.

_____

_____

Digestive System

Describe four ways in which tobacco use can affect the mouth and digestive system.

_____

_____

Circulatory System

What are four effects tobacco use has on the circulatory system?

_____

_____

Respiratory System

List four effects tobacco use can have on the respiratory system.

_____

_____

_____

Brain and Nervous System

Name two effects tobacco use has on the brain and nervous system.

_____

_____

Activity 43 — Applying Health Skills

Tobacco Use by the Numbers

The use of tobacco products is an expensive habit that affects millions of people. Although many people who use tobacco products want to quit, most are unable to kick the habit. The figures in the right column are statistics related to tobacco use in the United States. Match the descriptions in the left column with the appropriate statistic. Write the letter in the space provided.

_____ 1. Annual health care costs and lost productivity associated with tobacco use

_____ 2. Average cost per day of tobacco advertising and marketing campaigns

_____ 3. Approximate amount spent per year by people who smoke a pack of cigarettes a day

_____ 4. Approximate cost of one pack of cigarettes

_____ 5. Percentage of adults who do not use tobacco

_____ 6. Approximate number of former smokers, age 18 or older, in 1998

_____ 7. Number of people age 18 or older in 1998 who had never smoked

_____ 8. Decline in tobacco use among adults since 1965

a. $18.5 million

b. 75 percent

c. 40 percent

d. $1,000

e. 44 million

f. 103.8 million

g. $2.75

h. $100 billion

Answer the following questions about tobacco use. Write your answers on the lines provided.

9. Why do tobacco companies consider children and teens the most profitable market for their products?

_____

_____

10. Why do people who want to stop smoking find it difficult to do so?

_____

_____

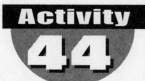

Applying Health Skills

Excuses, Excuses

Teen smokers give many excuses for their addiction. The truth is that there is no good reason to use tobacco. Here are some common excuses for smoking. On the lines after each one, write whether the influence that prompts the excuse is internal or external, which internal or external influence it is, and the fact about tobacco that makes the excuse invalid.

Excuse 1: "I smoke to keep my weight down so I can play sports."

Facts: _____

Excuse 2: "Smoking helps me relax when I need a break."

Facts: _____

_____

Excuse 3: "Why do I smoke? Because I want to! I'm independent! No one tells me what to do."

Facts: _____

_____

Excuse 4: "Smoking? What's the big deal? Everyone does it!"

Facts: _____

_____

Excuse 5: "My favorite actor always has a cigarette in photos."

Facts: _____

_____

Excuse 6: "Smoking makes me look cool."

Facts: _____

_____

Excuse 7: "Everyone smokes in movies. They wouldn't have famous actors smoking if it were bad for you."

Facts: _____

_____

Chapter **12** Health Inventory

The Truth About Tobacco

**Some of these statements about tobacco are true; some are false.
Identify each statement by writing *true* or *false* in the space at the left.**

_____ 1. Nonsmokers can be seriously harmed by secondhand smoke.

_____ 2. Cigar smokers are 4 to 10 times more likely to get cancer of the mouth and esophagus than nonsmokers.

_____ 3. Most smokers are satisfied with their addiction and don't want to quit.

_____ 4. Tobacco companies spend billions of dollars each year to get people to use their products.

_____ 5. Nicotine is a powerful drug and is more addictive than heroin or cocaine.

_____ 6. Women who smoke during pregnancy risk premature delivery or having a low-birth-weight baby.

_____ 7. Cigarette withdrawal symptoms include headaches, irritability, fatigue, and difficulty sleeping.

_____ 8. Burning tobacco produces carbon monoxide, which enters the bloodstream and reduces the amount of oxygen that the blood cells can carry.

_____ 9. Tobacco companies spend little money on advertising, since the product "sells itself."

_____ 10. Although it is physically addictive, tobacco is not psychologically addictive.

_____ 11. Tobacco use has no effect on public health costs or costs to the nation's economy.

_____ 12. The best way to maintain a tobacco-free life is never to start using tobacco products.

Score yourself:

Write the number of correct responses here.

10–12: Excellent

6–9: Fair

0–5: You're blinded by smoke! Don't believe the hype—learn the facts about tobacco.

Chapter 13 Study Guide

As you read the chapter, answer the following questions. Later you can use this guide to review the information in the chapter.

Lesson 1

1. List the long-term effects of alcohol on at least three parts of the body.

_____

_____

_____

_____

2. Identify four factors that determine the effect alcohol has on the drinker.

_____

_____

_____

3. Define *blood alcohol concentration (BAC)*, and identify the level at which a person is considered to be legally intoxicated.

_____

_____

4. Define *binge drinking*, and explain why it is especially dangerous.

_____

_____

_____

Lesson 2

5. Describe the effects of alcohol that makes it dangerous to drink and drive.

_____

6. Define *alcoholism*, and identify the three stages of alcoholism.

_____

_____

_____

_____

7. List three organizations that help alcoholics and their families.

_____

8. Identify two things you can do to help someone who has a drinking problem.

_____

_____

Lesson 3

9. What are three reasons teens might give for experimenting with alcohol?

_____

_____

_____

10. Give three reasons why an increasing number of young people are choosing not to drink.

_____

_____

_____

11. Give two alternatives to drinking.

_____

_____

_____

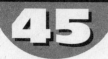

Activity 45

Applying Health Skills

Getting the Facts on Alcohol

Some of the statements below are facts; others are not. Classify each by writing *fact* or *myth* in the space at the left. On the lines that follow the statements, correct the ones you have identified as myths.

_____ 1. Drinking alcohol is not as dangerous as taking drugs.

_____

_____ 2. Alcohol causes perspiration to increase and skin to become flushed.

_____

_____ 3. Alcohol is a depressant that slows down the functions of the brain and other parts of the nervous system.

_____

_____ 4. Although it takes a long time, the brain can replace all the cells that are destroyed by alcohol.

_____

_____ 5. The same amount of alcohol has a greater effect on a small person than it does on a large one.

_____

_____ 6. Alcohol generally moves into the bloodstream faster in females.

_____

_____ 7. A BAC of less than .08 or .1 is legal for everyone.

_____

_____ 8. Two to three drinks can cause a loss of coordination and judgment.

_____

_____ 9. Fetal alcohol syndrome (FAS) is the leading known cause of mental retardation in the United States.

_____

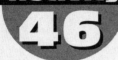

Activity 46

Applying Health Skills

Treatment for Alcoholism

People who become alcoholics develop their drinking problems over a period of time. Experts have identified three distinct stages of alcoholism.

Read the statements below. Identify the stage of alcoholism each statement describes by writing *1*, *2*, or *3* in the space at the left.

_____ 1. The drinker is often absent from school or work.

_____ 2. The drinker's body is strongly addicted to alcohol.

_____ 3. The body develops a need for more and more alcohol.

_____ 4. A person starts using alcohol to relax or to relieve stress.

_____ 5. The drinker begins to lie or make excuses about his or her drinking.

_____ 6. Drinking is out of control.

Answer the following questions about alcoholism. Write your answers on the lines provided.

7. How many families in the United States are affected by alcoholism?

_____

8. What effects can alcoholism have on a family?

_____

9. What are the four steps of the recovery process, and what do they involve?

_____

_____

_____

10. What are two support groups for families who are coping with alcoholism?

_____

_____

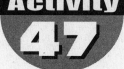

Activity 47

Use with Chapter 13, Lesson 3.

Applying Health Skills

Say No to Alcohol

Resisting peer pressure can be very difficult at times. Listed below are several ways to say no to alcohol. Complete the remaining sentences by suggesting other ways to refuse alcohol.

1. No, thanks, <u>drinking makes me sleepy.</u>

2. No, thanks, <u>I'm in training.</u>

3. No, thanks, <u>I don't like the taste.</u>

4. No, thanks, _____

5. No, thanks, _____

6. No, thanks, _____

7. No, thanks, _____

8. No, thanks, _____

9. No, thanks, _____

10. No, thanks, _____

11. No, thanks, _____

12. No, thanks, _____

13. No, thanks, _____

14. No, thanks, _____

15. No, thanks, _____

16. No, thanks, _____

17. No, thanks, _____

18. No, thanks, _____

19. No, thanks, _____

20. No, thanks!

Chapter 13 Health Inventory

Dealing with a Problem Drinker

Do you know someone who has a drinking problem? You may be able to help. Read each statement below. Circle *do* if you think it will help the drinker. Circle *don't* if you think it will not help.

do   don't   **1.** Talk calmly and honestly with the drinker about the harmful effects of alcohol.

do   don't   **2.** Argue with the drinker when he or she is drunk.

do   don't   **3.** Gather information about alcoholism.

do   don't   **4.** Threaten or bribe the drinker.

do   don't   **5.** Provide the drinker with information about organizations that help problem drinkers.

do   don't   **6.** Let the drinker know that his or her drinking worries you.

do   don't   **7.** Try to include the drinker in activities that do not involve alcohol.

do   don't   **8.** Allow the drinker to drive if the person thinks he or she can.

do   don't   **9.** Discuss the drinker's alcohol problem with a counselor or someone you trust.

do   don't   **10.** Encourage the drinker to seek help.

do   don't   **11.** Admit that a problem exists and try to get help.

do   don't   **12.** Encourage the drinker to feel confident about quitting.

do   don't   **13.** Ride with a driver who has been drinking.

do   don't   **14.** Learn as much as you can about alcoholism.

Score yourself:

Give yourself 4 points for each correct answer.

The *do's* are statements 1, 3, 5, 6, 7, 9, 10, 11, and 12.

The *don'ts* are statements 2, 4, 8, and 13.

48–56: Excellent; you have the knowledge to help someone with an alcohol problem.

32–44: Pretty good

Fewer than 32: Get the facts about alcoholism, and learn how you can help someone with a drinking problem.

Chapter 14 Study Guide

As you read the chapter, answer the following questions. Later you can use this guide to review the information in the chapter.

Lesson 1

1. List the skin's four basic functions.

_____

_____

2. Identify three important structures that are contained in the dermis.

_____

3. Explain why you should limit your exposure to direct sunlight.

_____

_____

4. Describe two problems that can affect the nails.

_____

_____

Lesson 2

5. Define *periodontium*, and explain what it does.

_____

_____

6. What is *plaque*, and how can it affect your teeth?

_____

_____

7. List four principles of sensible dental care.

_____

_____

Lesson 3

8. Name three parts of the eye, and explain what each does.

_____

_____

_____

_____

_____

9. Identify three ways you can protect your eyes.

_____

_____

_____

_____

10. Identify and describe one common vision problem.

_____

_____

_____

11. List four ways to take care of your ears.

_____

_____

_____

Activity 48

Applying Health Skills

Dear Dr. Skin Care

Imagine that you are a skin care expert. You write a magazine column for teens. Your job is to answer letters from readers who have questions about skin care. In today's mail you received the following three letters asking for advice. Carefully read each letter; then write a reply to each, telling the writer how to deal with his or her problem.

Letter 1

I have a problem. I have acne and I want to do something about it. What can I do to care for my skin?

_____

_____

_____

_____

Letter 2

Every article I read says something different about how to care for your skin. I'm confused about what to do to keep my skin healthy.

_____

_____

_____

_____

Letter 3

I like to go to the beach with my friends. In fact, we go to the beach just about every day during the summer. I have a nice tan, and everyone thinks I look great. However, I recently heard that spending too much time in the sun can cause premature aging of the skin and may lead to skin cancer. Is there anything I can do to avoid exposure to the sun and still spend time at the beach?

_____

_____

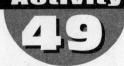

Activity 49

Applying Health Skills

Healthy Teeth

The Browns and the Greens are neighbors. Caring for their teeth is very important to one of these families. Find out which family is likely to have fewer dental problems by checking the items and habits that show healthy tooth care.

Brown Family

_____ Soft-bristled toothbrushes

_____ Toothpaste containing fluoride

_____ Dental floss

_____ All the Browns have had at least one dental checkup this year.

_____ The Brown children brush their teeth after every meal.

_____ The Browns limit sugar in their diets.

_____ The Browns replace their toothbrushes every two or three months.

_____ The Browns snack on raw fruits and vegetables.

_____ The Browns protect their teeth from injury when playing sports.

Green Family

_____ Hard toothbrushes

_____ Toothpaste containing fluoride

_____ No dental floss

_____ The Greens haven't gone to the dentist this year.

_____ The Green children brush their teeth only in the morning.

_____ The Greens brush the inner, outer, and chewing surfaces of their teeth.

_____ The Greens rely on mouthwash after meals to prevent tooth decay.

_____ The Greens eat lots of sugary snack foods.

_____ The Greens prefer chocolate or candy that remains in the mouth.

Count the number of checks each family has earned. Write those numbers here:

Brown Family _____   Green Family _____

On the lines that follow, list at least three changes the Greens should make to improve their dental care.

_____

_____

_____

Activity 50

Applying Health Skills

Taking Care of Your Eyes and Ears

Tell what you would do in each of the situations described below and explain why.

Situation 1

You have noticed that you are having a difficult time reading the chalkboard in your classes. What would you do? Why?

_____

_____

Situation 2

You are going to a rock concert.
What protection would you wear? Why?

_____

_____

Situation 3

Your sister has found some eye makeup in her drawer and isn't sure when she bought it. What would you tell her? Why?

_____

_____

Situation 4

You are going to spend all day tomorrow snowboarding.
What protection would you wear? Why?

_____

_____

Situation 5

You are going to have to spend several hours on your computer working on an essay. How would you prepare? Why?

_____

_____

Chapter **14** Health Inventory

Taking Stock

Here is a checklist to help you maintain your wellness and appearance. In the space at the left, put a check next to each item you do regularly.

_____   **1.** I bathe or shower daily.

_____   **2.** I brush my hair daily.

_____   **3.** I use a fluoride toothpaste.

_____   **4.** I wear comfortable, well-fitting shoes.

_____   **5.** I use protective eyewear when I need it.

_____   **6.** I keep foreign objects out of my ears.

_____   **7.** I play the radio, stereo, and TV at a reasonable volume.

_____   **8.** I use a sunscreen with an SPF of 15 or higher for all outdoor activities.

_____   **9.** I visit the dentist regularly.

_____   **10.** I allow my hair to air-dry.

_____   **11.** I avoid sugary snacks.

_____   **12.** I floss my teeth regularly.

_____   **13.** I rest my eyes periodically.

_____   **14.** I cut my toenails straight across.

_____   **15.** I protect my ears in cold weather.

Score yourself:

How many items did you check? Write that number here.

11–15: Wellness and appearance are very important to you.

6–10: Wellness and appearance are somewhat important to you.

Fewer than 6: You will look and feel better if you change some of your habits.

Chapter 15 Study Guide

> **STUDY TIPS**
> ✔ Read the chapter objectives.
> ✔ Look up any unfamiliar words.
> ✔ Read the questions below before you read the chapter.

As you read the chapter, answer the following questions. Later you can use this guide to review the information in the chapter.

Lesson 1

1. Name three kinds of joints, and give an example of each.

_____

_____

2. Identify two types of connective tissue and their functions.

_____

_____

Lesson 2

3. Identify the three types of muscle tissue and the jobs they do.

_____

_____

_____

Lesson 3

4. Describe two of the three main types of blood vessels and what they do.

_____

_____

_____

5. Identify four parts of the blood.

_____

Lesson 4

6. Name five parts of the respiratory system.

_____

7. List three disorders of the respiratory system.

_____

_____

Lesson 5

8. List two safety rules for preventing head and spinal cord injuries.

_____

_____

Lesson 6

9. Name four problems of the digestive system.

_____

_____

Lesson 7

10. Describe the functions of the thyroid and adrenal glands.

_____

_____

_____

Lesson 8

11. Name two tasks of the female reproductive system.

_____

_____

Activity 51 Applying Health Skills

The Skeletal System

From the list at the right, choose the bones found in the parts of the body listed on the left. Then identify each type of skeletal system problem described at the bottom, using the terms listed in the box.

Arms _____

Legs _____

Feet _____

Hands _____

| |
| femur |
| metacarpals |
| humerus |
| patella |
| carpals |
| radius |
| phalanges |
| ulna |
| fibula |
| tarsals |
| tibia |
| metatarsals |

_____ **1.** The swelling of a joint because of stretched or twisted ligaments

_____ **2.** A curvature of the spine

_____ **3.** A break or crack in a bone caused by an injury

_____ **4.** Swollen and stiff joints caused by a breakdown of cartilage and wear and tear on joints

_____ **5.** A bone pushed out of its joint

_____ **6.** Brittle, porous bones, often caused by lack of calcium

| |
| **a.** osteoarthritis |
| **b.** scoliosis |
| **c.** fracture |
| **d.** dislocation |
| **e.** osteoporosis |
| **f.** sprain |

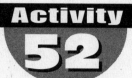

Applying Health Skills

Use with Chapter 15, Lesson 2.

Muscular System Injuries

Read the paragraph below about some common injuries to the muscular system. Then answer the questions that follow.

Many sports injuries occur at the beginning of an athletic season or when a person begins exercising after a long period of inactivity. In most cases these injuries require little treatment other than rest. However, a recurring injury may mean giving up the activity. An injury that recurs may lead to permanent damage.

Common muscle injuries include the following: A *strained muscle* occurs when a muscle is overused. The symptoms are pain and swelling. An ice pack applied to the affected area will reduce the pain and swelling. *Shin splints*, pain in the front of the lower legs, result from repeated straining of the muscles between the shin bones. In most cases the symptoms are treated by resting the muscles for a week or two. A *cramp* is a painful spasm, or tightening, in a muscle. An ordinary cramp lasts a few minutes and will clear up on its own. One can ease the discomfort by massaging and stretching the muscle and by applying heat.

1. Contrast a muscle cramp and a muscle strain.

2. Identify the treatment most often recommended for muscle injuries.

3. Explain why an ice pack is used to treat a muscle strain.

4. What causes shin splints?

5. List three ways to ease the discomfort of a muscle cramp.

Activity 53

Applying Health Skills

The Circulatory System

Imagine that you work in a health clinic that specializes in diagnosing and preventing heart problems. Read the questions that people might ask about the circulatory system. Write your response.

1. What is blood? What does it consist of?

   _____

   _____

2. If I need to have a transfusion, how do I know that the blood I would receive is safe?

   _____

   _____

   _____

3. Why is monitoring my blood pressure so important?

   _____

   _____

4. Why can it be dangerous to receive blood of a type that is different from your own?

   _____

   _____

5. The doctor says I have a problem with a pulmonary artery. What does this artery do?

   _____

   _____

6. What can I do to keep my heart strong and healthy and increase my chances of living a long and healthy life?

   _____

   _____

Activity 54 Applying Health Skills

The Respiratory System

Imagine that you are on a quiz show. One of the categories is the human respiratory system. The quiz show host presents an answer. You have to write a question.

1. Answer: You would not be able to eat without having this flap of tissue cover your trachea when you swallow.

   Question: _____

2. Answer: It's here that oxygen is transferred to the blood and carbon dioxide is removed.

   Question: _____

3. Answer: These are microscopic air sacs in the lungs where carbon dioxide is exchanged with oxygen.

   Question: _____

4. Answer: This disease, in which alveoli are damaged or destroyed, causes serious breathing difficulties.

   Question: _____

5. Answer: These two respiratory problems are strongly linked to smoking.

   Question: _____

6. Answer: This passage, also called the windpipe, directs air to the lungs.

   Question: _____

7. Answer: This is where air enters and leaves the body.

   Question: _____

8. Answer: This large dome-shaped muscle separates the lungs from the abdomen.

   Question: _____

Activity 55 — Applying Health Skills

The Nervous System

Complete the diagram below by labeling the three main parts of the brain and describing the function of each. Then answer the questions below.

a. _____

_____

b. _____

c. _____

_____

d. _____

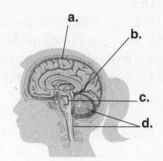

1. What are the two main parts of the nervous system, and what does each include?

_____

_____

2. Identify two types of involuntary actions and two types of voluntary actions controlled by the central nervous system.

_____

3. What are the two main parts of the peripheral nervous system, and what is the function of each?

_____

4. Name three diseases unrelated to injuries that can affect the nervous system.

_____

5. What are *neurons*, and what is their function?

_____

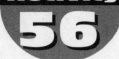

Applying Health Skills

Caring for Your Digestive and Excretory Systems

Below is a list of important Do's and Don'ts for your digestive system. Read the DO list to find out what you should do to care for your digestive system. Read the DON'T list to learn what to avoid.

DO
- Eat a variety of foods.
- Eat complete meals.
- Take time to relax and enjoy meals.
- Chew food thoroughly.

DON'T
- Forget to drink plenty of water.
- Skip meals.
- Rush through your meal.
- Try to wash large pieces of food down with a beverage.

During the next three days, try to practice the Do's listed above and avoid the Don'ts. Monitor yourself three times a day—morning, afternoon, and evening. Use the chart below to show your progress. Write an *A* in the chart for each Do you practice during that part of the day, and write an *X* for each Don't.

	DAY 1	DAY 2	DAY 3
Morning			
Afternoon			
Evening			

At the end of three days, add the total number of *A*s and *X*s. Write these numbers below.

Number of *A*s: _____   Number of *X*s: _____

If there are more *A*s than *X*s, give yourself a reward. If there are more *X*s than *A*s, list three ways you can improve the care of your digestive system.

_____

_____

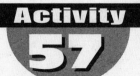

Activity 57

Applying Health Skills

Your Endocrine System

The diagram below shows the glands of the endocrine system. Identify each gland by writing its name on the line provided.

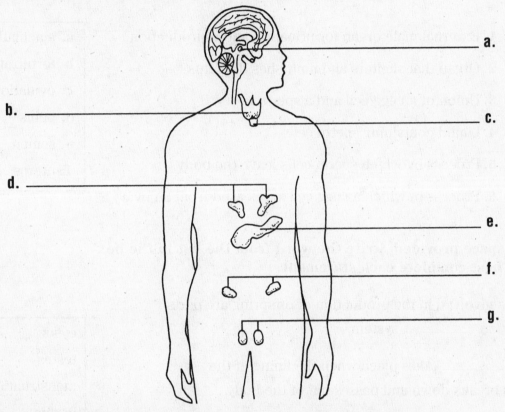

a. _____

b. _____

c. _____

d. _____

e. _____

f. _____

g. _____

Below is a list of the jobs glands do. Match each job with the correct gland from the diagram. Write the letter of the gland in the space provided.

_____ 1. Produces insulin and contains cells that control blood sugar levels

_____ 2. Reproduction in males

_____ 3. Regulates the chemical reactions of nutrients in the cells

_____ 4. Signals other glands to produce hormones when needed

_____ 5. Reproduction in females

_____ 6. Controls the body's response to emergencies

_____ 7. Directs the distribution of certain minerals in the body

Activity 58   Applying Health Skills

The Reproductive System

Match each definition in the left column with the correct term from the right column. Write the letter of the term in the space provided.

_____ 1. External male organ for urination and reproduction

_____ 2. Organ that shelters and nourishes the fetus

_____ 3. Union of an egg cell and a sperm cell

_____ 4. Liquid containing sperm cells

_____ 5. Process by which sperm cells leave the body

_____ 6. Process in which an egg cell is released from an ovary

> **a.** ejaculation
> **b.** fertilization
> **c.** ovulation
> **d.** penis
> **e.** semen
> **f.** uterus

In the space provided, write the word from the list in the box that will best complete each statement.

7. Organs involved in the production of offspring are parts of the _____ system.

8. _____ takes place when the lining of the uterus breaks down and passes out of the body.

9. Ovarian _____ are growths on the ovary.

10. The glands that produce sperm are called the _____.

11. Sperm mature and are stored temporarily in the _____.

12. A _____ is a male reproductive cell.

13. _____ is the inability of females to reproduce.

14. The sequence of events that occurs from one menstruation to the next is the menstrual _____.

15. An inguinal _____ is a tissue separation that allows part of the intestine to push into the scrotum.

> cysts
> testes
> menstruation
> hernia
> cycle
> infertility
> sperm
> reproductive
> epididymis

Chapter 15 Health Inventory

Taking Care of the Systems of Your Body

Here is a list of guidelines to help you care for the various systems of your body. In the spaces at the left, write *yes* for the guidelines you follow and *no* for those you do not follow.

_____ 1. Get plenty of rest.

_____ 2. Eat balanced meals that are high in fiber and low in fat.

_____ 3. Drink plenty of water.

_____ 4. Sit, stand, and walk with straight posture.

_____ 5. Avoid the use of drugs, alcohol, and tobacco.

_____ 6. Obey all traffic safety rules.

_____ 7. Wear protective equipment when bicycling, skating, or playing a contact sport.

_____ 8. Avoid situations where a blow to the head could occur.

_____ 9. Wear a safety belt whenever you are in a car.

_____ 10. Lift objects properly, and do not lift more than you can carry.

_____ 11. Keep your weight at a level that is healthy for you.

_____ 12. Engage in regular physical activity.

_____ 13. Reduce your level of stress when you can.

_____ 14. Have regular dental examinations.

_____ 15. Bathe or shower daily.

Score yourself:

Write the number of *yes* answers here.

12–15: Congratulations! You understand the importance of caring for your body systems.

8–11: Come on! Work a little harder.

Fewer than 8: Warning! This is the only body you'll ever have; take care of it.

Chapter 16 Study Guide

As you read the chapter, answer the following questions. Later you can use this guide to review the information in the chapter.

Lesson 1

1. Define *cells*, *tissues*, *organs*, and *systems*.

_____

_____

2. Explain what *fertilization* is.

_____

_____

3. Explain the difference between an *embryo* and a *fetus*.

_____

_____

4. Explain what the *placenta* and the *umbilical cord* do.

_____

_____

Lesson 2

5. Define *chromosomes* and *genes*.

_____

_____

6. Name two types of genetic disorders.

7. Identify four environmental factors that can contribute to birth defects.

Lesson 3

8. List the eight stages of development identified by scientist Erik Erikson.

9. List three developmental tasks of adolescence.

10. Identify three physical changes that occur in both males and females during puberty.

Lesson 4

11. Identify and describe three different ways to measure age.

12. List three ways to make aging a more positive experience.

Activity 59

Applying Health Skills

A New Life

Write the correct title from the list below on each numbered answer line. Then number the steps in each lettered list in the correct order.

Titles: The Birth Process
Fertilization and Early Growth
Fetal Development

1. _____

_____ a. The fertilized cluster of cells attaches itself to the wall of the uterus.

_____ b. The placenta begins to provide nourishment to the developing fetus.

_____ c. The fertilized cell begins to divide.

_____ d. A sperm cell joins with an egg cell.

2. _____

_____ a. The heart, brain, and lungs begin to form.

_____ b. The arms and legs can move freely.

_____ c. The heart is beating.

_____ d. Body organs have developed to function on their own.

3. _____

_____ a. Contractions push the placenta out of the mother's body.

_____ b. Mild contractions begin.

_____ c. The cervix opens to a width of about 4 inches.

_____ d. The baby is born.

Activity 60

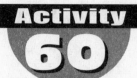

Use with Chapter 16, Lesson 2.

Applying Health Skills

Dominant or Recessive?

You have learned that genes determine which traits of your parents get passed along to you. Each parent supplies one gene. Some genes are *dominant*. Others are *recessive*. The dominant gene is the stronger one. This means that if you inherit the dominant brown hair gene from one parent and the recessive blond hair gene from the other, you will have brown hair.

This activity allows you to look at some other traits that you have inherited and discover whether you have dominant traits or recessive traits. Read the paragraphs below and complete the chart that follows.

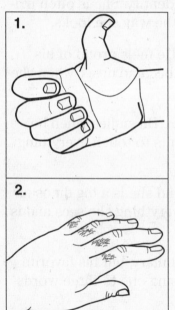

1. Try bending your thumb back. Some people can bend the last joint of the thumb back beyond an angle of 45°, as seen in the picture to the left. This is called hitchhiker's thumb. If you cannot bend your thumb more than 45°, you have the dominant gene *L*. If you can bend your thumb more than 45°, you have the recessive gene *l*. Circle the appropriate letter, *L* or *l*, on the chart.

2. Look at the back of your hand. Examine the first segment of each finger for the presence of hair. In some cases there may be no hair present. In other cases there may be hair on all four fingers, or in still other cases, there may be hair on one, two, or three fingers. See the hair on the fingers in the drawing at the left. If there is any hair at all on the first segment of your fingers, you have the dominant gene *H*. Circle the appropriate letter, *H* or *h*, on the chart.

3. Another trait that you have inherited is a tendency toward right-handedness or left-handedness. Right-handedness (*R*) is dominant over left-handedness (*r*). Circle the appropriate letter, *R* or *r*, on the chart.

My Inherited Traits		
Trait	Visible Characteristics	
1. Thumb Bending	Less than 45° L	More than 45° I
2. Finger Hair	Hair H	No hair h
3. Right- or Left- Handedness	Right-handed R	Left-handed r

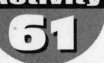

Activity 61

Use with Chapter 16, Lesson 3.

Applying Health Skills

The Stages of Growth

Even though everyone grows at a slightly different rate, each individual passes through certain stages of development. Read the description of each person below. Identify the developmental stage by writing *I* for infancy, *E* for early childhood, *M* for middle childhood, *L* for late childhood, or *A* for adolescence.

_____ 1. Eric has recently developed a great interest in model cars. After many tries he has successfully put together a model car from a kit.

_____ 2. Samantha is beginning to develop a sense of her own identity. She is often irritated for no reason. However, she is beginning to like the way she looks.

_____ 3. Brian has just learned to climb the stairs in his home. He feels proud of his achievement but does not understand why his mother became upset when she saw him working his way up to the top step alone.

_____ 4. Toshio is beginning to recognize the people around him. He smiles when he sees his mother's face and laughs when tickled. He wants to touch everything he can reach.

_____ 5. Andrea would rather run than walk. She loves to pretend she is a big dinosaur that growls and chases people. She is curious about everything she sees and is constantly asking her parents, "Why?"

_____ 6. Ben has recently added several new words to his vocabulary, but his favorite word is still *no*. He is able to ask for what he wants, using one to three words at a time.

_____ 7. Carlos is teased by his family for his cracking, changing voice, and he thinks it is funny, too. He has applied for a part-time job after school. If he gets it, he looks forward to proving he can keep up with both his job and his schoolwork.

_____ 8. Lo has started following her father around the house and imitating what he does. She wants to help him do everything, so he bought her a set of play tools to use while he works on his own projects.

_____ 9. In the last few months Caroline has begun to hear the rhythms in music and to follow along with real dance steps. She has learned almost every dance her older sister has taught her.

Activity 62   Applying Health Skills

Growing Older and Staying Well

After we become adults, we pass through three basic stages in the aging process: early adulthood, middle adulthood, and late adulthood. Each stage is marked by certain milestones, and how well we age depends on a variety of physical, mental and emotional, and physical factors.

Complete the charts below by identifying some of these milestones and factors. Then answer the questions that follow.

Stage of Adulthood	Milestones
Early Adulthood	
Middle Adulthood	
Late Adulthood	

Health Triangle	Factors that can affect aging
Physical Health	
Mental/Emotional Health	
Social Health	

1. In what ways may people follow the stages of adulthood in a less predictable sequence?

_____

_____

_____

2. What are three different ways in which age can be measured?

_____

_____

3. Why is it important for adults to pay attention to all three sides of the health triangle?

_____

Chapter 16 Health Inventory

Becoming an Adult

Read the statements below. In the space at the left, write *yes* if the statement describes you, or *no* if it does not describe you.

_____   **1.** I am preparing now for the responsibilities and challenges of adulthood.

_____   **2.** I think it is important to be involved in the community even though I am still in my teen years.

_____   **3.** I am beginning to think about the type of work I am interested in doing after I finish school.

_____   **4.** I get my assignments done on time.

_____   **5.** I can make my own decisions without giving in to peer pressure.

_____   **6.** I carry out my responsibilities without being reminded.

_____   **7.** My behavior reflects my personal standards and values.

_____   **8.** I know what people like and dislike about me.

_____   **9.** I understand that my actions affect other people.

_____   **10.** I believe that elderly people have the same emotional needs as younger people do.

_____   **11.** The health habits I have now will help me live a long and healthy life.

_____   **12.** I expect to be mentally and physically active throughout my life.

_____   **13.** I am good at accepting changes in my life.

_____   **14.** I expect to work for what I want rather than just have things happen to me.

_____   **15.** I think that my chances of reaching my goals for the future are good.

Score yourself:

Write the number of *yes* answers here.

12–15: Excellent

8–11: Good

Fewer than 8: Adolescence is a time to begin taking more responsibility for your actions. How can you improve in this area?

Chapter 17 Study Guide

   As you read the chapter, answer the following questions. Later you can use this guide to review the information in the chapter.

Lesson 1

1. Identify three types of pathogens that cause communicable diseases.

_____

2. List four ways pathogens can be spread.

_____

_____

3. Identify two ways to prevent the spread of communicable diseases.

_____

_____

_____

_____

Lesson 2

4. List the body's first line of defenses against disease.

_____

5. Name the two major kinds of defense strategies of the body's immune system.

_____

_____

6. Explain how vaccines help your body fight disease.

_____

_____

Lesson 3

7. Name two of the most common communicable diseases.

_____

8. List three good health habits that can reduce your chances of illness.

_____

Lesson 4

9. List three important facts about sexually transmitted infections (STIs).

_____

_____

_____

_____

10. Name three of the most serious common STIs, and tell how they can be prevented.

_____

_____

Lesson 5

11. Describe what effect HIV has on a person's immune system.

_____

_____

12. List three ways HIV can be spread.

_____

_____

Activity 63 Applying Health Skills

Preventing Communicable Diseases

There are many ways of helping to prevent the spread of communicable diseases. Read the following situations. Write what is wrong with each situation below and what the person should do differently in order to guard against disease.

Situation 1

Brittany's sister had had a bad cold for several days. Brittany brought a new box of tissues to the kitchen, where her sister was drinking a glass of orange juice. "Can I have a sip of your juice?" Brittany asked.

_____

_____

Situation 2

At the picnic, Max could not wait to have some of the barbecued chicken. When he bit into a piece, he noticed that the bone was still pink and there was some blood in the tissues. However, he was so hungry that he continued eating.

_____

_____

Situation 3

The day was getting hotter. Even though Carly was wearing shorts and a T-shirt, she was quite warm. She decided to cut through the densely forested, shady lot between the road and her home because it was cooler than the road.

_____

_____

Situation 4

Tom wondered how long his flu would last. He still did not feel well, but he wanted to go to school anyway. He asked his mother to cancel the doctor's appointment she had made. Then he got ready for school.

_____

_____

Activity 64

Use with Chapter 17, Lesson 2.

Applying Health Skills

Defending the Body Against Infection

The body has three main layers of defense against possible invading pathogens. Complete the following chart to show these layers of defense.

Defense	Body Systems	How Pathogens Are Repelled
first line of defense		
nonspecific response		
specific response		

Activity 65

Use with Chapter 17, Lesson 3.

Applying Health Skills

Communicable Diseases Chart

Below is a list of some communicable diseases. Complete as much of the chart as possible by filling in the symptoms and contagious period for each.

Disease	Symptoms	Contagious Period
chicken pox		
rubella		
pneumonia		
tuberculosis		
Lyme disease		

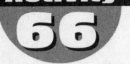

Activity 66　Applying Health Skills

Use with Chapter 17, Lesson 4.

Facts on Sexually Transmitted Infections

Information is one of the most important defenses in the prevention of sexually transmitted infections (STIs). To check your knowledge, answer the questions below.

1. How great is the risk of getting STIs for teens ages 15 to 19?

_____

2. What are some permanent conditions that can result from untreated STIs?

_____

3. Why are people often not aware that they have an STI?

_____

4. What can people who get an STI do in order to have the best chance of being cured?

_____

5. What is the only sure way to avoid getting any STI?

_____

6. Which STI affects only women?

_____

7. Which STI can cause blindness, insanity, paralysis, and death?

_____

8. Painful blisters in the genital area are possible signs of what kind of STI?

_____

9. How do STIs differ from other communicable diseases?

_____

10. What are two reasons to feel good about choosing abstinence from sexual activity?

_____

Activity 67 — Applying Health Skills

AIDS Facts and Myths

Some of the statements below are facts; others are not. Classify each by writing *fact* or *myth* on the line at the left.

_____ 1. HIV attacks and weakens the body's immune system.

_____ 2. Piercing the skin with contaminated needles can spread HIV.

_____ 3. Unborn babies can get HIV from their mothers.

_____ 4. You can get HIV by using the same eating utensils as an infected person.

_____ 5. There is no cure for AIDS.

_____ 6. People can catch HIV from infected mosquitoes.

_____ 7. One way to get HIV is to give blood.

_____ 8. Carriers can spread HIV even though they show no signs of the virus themselves.

_____ 9. You cannot tell if someone has HIV by his or her appearance.

_____ 10. Being infected with HIV makes it possible for other pathogens to attack the body.

_____ 11. Shaking hands with a person who is infected with HIV can spread the disease.

_____ 12. One way to get HIV is to touch something an infected person has touched.

Imagine that you are in charge of publicizing the facts about HIV/AIDS. On the lines below, list three actions you would take to get the facts to the public.

_____

_____

_____

Preventing the Spread of Disease

Making the right choices can decrease your chances of catching and spreading diseases. For each item below, circle the word that shows how often you behave as described.

always	usually	sometimes	1. I get enough sleep every night.
always	usually	sometimes	2. I follow a sensible eating plan.
always	usually	sometimes	3. I make sure that food is properly stored and cooked.
always	usually	sometimes	4. I use clean utensils and preparation surfaces when I prepare food.
always	usually	sometimes	5. I do not share drinking glasses or utensils with anyone else.
always	usually	sometimes	6. I wash my hands before eating or handling food.
always	usually	sometimes	7. I avoid alcohol and drugs.
always	usually	sometimes	8. I keep my vaccinations current against diseases such as polio, tetanus, and measles.
always	usually	sometimes	9. I cover my mouth when I cough or sneeze.
always	usually	sometimes	10. I seek treatment right away if I think I might be ill.
always	usually	sometimes	11. If I am contagious, I stay home until I am better.
always	usually	sometimes	12. I exercise regularly.
always	usually	sometimes	13. I avoid tobacco.
always	usually	sometimes	14. I abstain from sexual activity.
always	usually	sometimes	15. I do not share personal items, such as towels, with others.

Score yourself:

Give yourself 5 points for each *always* answer, 3 points for each *usually*, and 1 point for each *sometimes*. Write your score here.

60–75: Your disease prevention measures are very good.

40–59: You practice some preventive habits but could do more.

Fewer than 40: Watch out! You need to practice more careful prevention.

Chapter **18** Study Guide

   As you read the chapter, answer the following questions. Later you can use this guide to review the information in the chapter.

Lesson 1

1. Explain the difference between *communicable* and *noncommunicable diseases*.

_____

_____

_____

2. Identify six common noncommunicable diseases.

_____

_____

3. List three habits that help prevent lifestyle diseases.

_____

_____

Lesson 2

4. Identify three common allergens.

_____

_____

5. Name three ways in which allergens enter the body.

_____

Lesson 3

6. Explain how the two kinds of tumors are different.

_____

7. List at least five of the seven warning signs of cancer.

_____

_____

_____

Lesson 4

8. Define *arteriosclerosis* and *atherosclerosis*.

_____

_____

9. Name four treatment options for heart and circulatory problems.

_____

_____

10. Identify four risk factors that can increase a person's risk of developing heart and circulatory problems.

_____

_____

Lesson 5

11. Describe the two types of diabetes.

_____

_____

12. List two ways to reduce the risk of developing type 2 diabetes.

_____

_____

Activity 68 · Applying Health Skills

The Truth About Noncommunicable Diseases

Some of the following statements about noncommunicable diseases are facts; others are not. Classify each statement by writing *true* or *false* in the space at the left. On the lines that follow the statements, correct the ones you have identified as false.

_____ 1. Noncommunicable diseases can be spread through contact with another person.

_____

_____

_____ 2. Cardiovascular diseases affect the heart and blood vessels.

_____

_____

_____ 3. Lifestyle behaviors have little effect on the incidence of noncommunicable diseases.

_____

_____

_____ 4. Tobacco use is a cause of respiratory and heart diseases and cancer.

_____

_____

_____ 5. Damage to the brain that results in cerebral palsy can occur before birth.

_____

_____

_____ 6. Little can be done to help people who are born with genetic disorders or birth defects.

_____

_____

_____ 7. Various environmental substances, such as chemical wastes and secondhand smoke, can cause serious health problems or make existing health problems worse.

_____

_____

Activity 69

Applying Health Skills

Understanding Allergies and Asthma

Identify each term in the right column by matching it with the correct description in the left column. Write the letter of the term in the space provided.

_____ 1. substances that can cause an allergic reaction

_____ 2. chemicals in the body that cause the symptoms of an allergic reaction

_____ 3. raised bumps on the skin that are very itchy

_____ 4. medicines that help control the effect of the chemicals that cause allergic reactions

_____ 5. a serious chronic condition that causes air passages in the respiratory system to become narrow or blocked

_____ 6. medicines used to relax muscles that have tightened around airways

> **a.** antihistamines
> **b.** bronchodilators
> **c.** allergens
> **d.** histamines
> **e.** hives
> **f.** asthma

Answer the following questions about allergies and asthma. Write your answers on the lines provided.

7. What are the three ways in which allergy-causing substances enter the body?

_____

8. How does the respiratory system usually respond to an allergen?

_____

9. What are four common asthma triggers?

_____

_____

10. How can people cope with asthma?

_____

_____

Activity 70

Applying Health Skills

Understanding Cancer

Read the descriptions below. On the lines following each description, identify and explain a cancer risk for each person and what the person might do to reduce the risk.

The Great Outdoors

Lori has fair skin and light-blond hair. Her favorite sports are hiking, surfing, and swimming in the ocean.

1. What form of cancer might Lori be at risk for? Why?

_____

_____

2. What can she do to reduce this risk?

_____

_____

A Problem Diet

Geraldo's favorite dinner is a hamburger and french fries. His other choices are fried chicken and buttered potatoes, or spaghetti and sausage. He eats vegetables and fruit about once a week.

3. What form of cancer might Geraldo be at risk for?

_____

4. What can he do to reduce this risk?

_____

Up in Smoke

Roy has been smoking about a pack of cigarettes a day for eight years.

5. What form of cancer might Roy be at risk for? Why?

_____

6. What can he do to reduce this risk?

_____

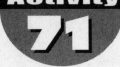

Activity 71

Use with Chapter 18, Lesson 4.

Applying Health Skills

Preventing Heart Disease

The following are completed profiles of two patients at a doctor's office. Decide whether each patient is at risk for heart problems by writing an *X* before each item that describes a risk factor. Then answer the questions.

Patient A, 35 years old

_____ has recently completed a course on stress management at work

_____ maintains a healthy weight

_____ has a family history of high blood pressure

_____ has not had a medical checkup in four years

_____ engages in regular physical activity

_____ has made an effort to reduce the amount of fat he eats

_____ does not smoke

_____ is a heavy alcohol drinker

Patient B, 45 years old

_____ is about 30 pounds overweight

_____ has regular medical checkups

_____ recently started a high-stress job

_____ has no family history of high blood pressure or heart disease

_____ eats foods that are fairly high in fat and low in fiber

_____ rarely has time for physical activity

_____ smokes about a pack of cigarettes a day

_____ rarely drinks alcohol

Count the number of checks in each patient profile. Write it here.

Patient A _____   Patient B _____

1. Which patient is more likely to develop heart problems?

_____

2. What lifestyle improvements could Patient A make?

_____

_____

3. What lifestyle improvements could Patient B make?

_____

_____

Activity 72

Applying Health Skills

Relief for Arthritis Sufferers

Read the paragraphs below, and answer the questions that follow.

The pain and stiffness of a joint can prevent a person with arthritis from doing even the simplest things, such as getting out of bed or walking. In the past, people with arthritis could hope for only temporary relief from the pain by use of medication. Today doctors can replace a diseased hip or knee with a prosthetic, or artificial, joint. These prosthetic devices have the same basic parts as a natural hip or knee.

An orthopedic surgeon—a doctor specializing in bone and joint surgery— determines whether or not replacement surgery is right for the patient. The doctor takes X-rays to see the degree of damage in the joint. Then the doctor does an examination to see how much motion the patient has lost in the affected joint.

The actual surgery takes several hours. After a few days of bed rest, physical therapy begins. This therapy consists of gentle exercises to strengthen the muscles around the new joint. As soon as possible, the patient is helped to use the replaced joint. The patient continues the exercises at home. After a few weeks the doctor will want to see the patient for a follow-up examination. At that time the doctor will test the patient's range of motion in the new joint.

1. Explain how a prosthetic joint is similar to a normal hip or knee.

_____

2. Identify the body parts on which orthopedic surgeons perform surgery.

_____

3. List three steps in the recovery from joint replacement surgery.

_____

4. Why do you think the orthopedic surgeon tests the patient's range of motion both before and after the surgery?

_____

5. Contrast arthritis treatment in the past with arthritis treatment today.

_____

Chapter **18** Health Inventory

An Ounce of Prevention

Do you follow the good health habits that will help protect you from getting noncommunicable diseases? Use the questions below to find out. Write *yes* or *no* in the space at the left of each statement.

_____ **1.** Do you limit the amount of fat you eat?

_____ **2.** Do you limit the amount of salt you eat?

_____ **3.** Do you eat plenty of whole grains, fruits, and vegetables?

_____ **4.** Do you know the warning signs of melanoma?

_____ **5.** Do you maintain a healthy weight?

_____ **6.** Do you engage in regular physical activity?

_____ **7.** Do you get plenty of rest?

_____ **8.** Do you deal well with stress in your daily life?

_____ **9.** Do you avoid using tobacco?

_____ **10.** Do you avoid using alcohol?

_____ **11.** Do you avoid using drugs?

_____ **12.** Do you use sunscreens to protect your skin from the sun?

_____ **13.** Do you perform regular self-examinations for breast or testicular cancer?

_____ **14.** Do you watch for the seven warning signs of cancer?

_____ **15.** Do you know your family's medical history?

Score yourself:

Write the number of *yes* answers here.

12–15: Good for you! You're taking good care of yourself.

8–11: Fair; you can do better.

Fewer than 8: You are in trouble. Remember, only a healthy body can fight disease.

Chapter **19** Study Guide

   As you read the chapter, answer the following questions. Later you can use this guide to review the information in the chapter.

Lesson 1

1. List three guidelines to follow to act safely.

_____

2. Define the *accident chain*, and explain how it can be broken.

_____

_____

Lesson 2

3. List three traffic safety rules that people should follow.

_____

_____

4. List three safety guidelines to follow when hiking or camping.

_____

_____

Lesson 3

5. Identify three actions you should take to prepare for a hurricane.

_____

_____

6. List two actions you should take if an earthquake strikes while you are inside a building.

_____

_____

Lesson 4

7. Name the sequence of steps to follow in an emergency situation.

_____

8. Describe the type of care you should provide to a victim of injury while waiting for help to arrive.

_____

_____

_____

_____

Lesson 5

9. Describe the correct procedure for removing ticks.

_____

_____

_____

10. Describe the three types of burns.

_____

_____

_____

Lesson 6

11. Define *shock*, and list signs of shock.

_____

_____

_____

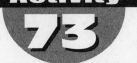

Activity 73 Applying Health Skills

Who Is Safety Conscious?

Read the statements below. Write *safe* on the line at the left if the statement describes a safety-conscious person. Write *unsafe* if the statement describes a person who is not safety conscious. Change each unsafe behavior to a safe one on the line following the statement.

_____ **1.** Diana is alert to possible hazards around her.

_____

_____ **2.** Morgan often acts on impulse instead of planning ahead.

_____

_____ **3.** Gus uses a step stool or ladder when trying to reach high places.

_____

_____ **4.** Jerry almost never cleans his stove, even when he spills food on it.

_____

_____ **5.** Andrea makes a point of being more careful when she's tired or upset.

_____

_____ **6.** Melinda sometimes acts recklessly to impress her peers.

_____

_____ **7.** Leah tries to call attention to herself by taking unnecessary risks.

_____

_____ **8.** Tom knows what to do in case of a fire in his home.

_____

_____ **9.** Wes stores a loaded gun in his unlocked closet.

_____

_____ **10.** Felicia takes responsibility for her own safety.

_____

Activity 74

Applying Health Skills

Safety Check

Read the statements below. Identify each safe statement by writing *S* in the space at the left, and each unsafe statement by writing *U*.

_____ 1. Martin seldom uses his safety belt when he drives his car.

_____ 2. Moira wears a helmet whenever she rides her bike, even if she is just riding around the block near her house.

_____ 3. Alan always crosses streets at the designated crosswalks.

_____ 4. Bill and Ed agree to stay together during their hike up Bear Mountain.

_____ 5. Brent is shivering in the cold rain, but he decides to continue jogging for another half hour.

_____ 6. Although a thunderstorm is starting and she can see lightning, Pam continues to swim in the lake.

_____ 7. Before the rest of Ann's family gets up each morning, she exercises by swimming alone across Lily Lake.

_____ 8. Rowena dresses for a cold day outside by wearing several layers of clothing.

_____ 9. Edwin hears someone calling for help from the deep end of the pool, so he jumps in to try to help even though he is not a strong swimmer himself.

_____ 10. Marina and Sandy dare each other to eat the berries of the plants they find along a hiking trail.

_____ 11. Jeanette often rides a bicycle on the road at night without wearing reflective clothing or having reflectors on her bike.

_____ 12. Brad and George ignore the "Thin Ice" signs because they want to practice ice hockey on the lake. The signs have been posted most of the winter.

_____ 13. Before leaving the campsite, Stacy pours water on the glowing embers of her campfire and also covers it with dirt.

_____ 14. Mike continues to use his skateboard even though he has lost his helmet.

_____ 15. Although Gary has been skiing only once before, he agrees to try the expert slope with two of his friends, both of whom are excellent skiers.

_____ 16. Before Rick dives into the lake, he checks the depth of the water.

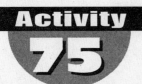

Activity 75

Applying Health Skills

What Would You Do?

On the lines provided, tell what you would do in each weather emergency described below.

Situation 1
You are at home listening to the radio when a tornado warning is announced.
What would you do?

_____

_____

Situation 2
The National Weather Service has issued a hurricane warning for your area. You are the only person at home, and you have been unable to reach older family members by telephone.
What would you do?

_____

_____

Situation 3
You are outdoors when a winter snowstorm unexpectedly turns into a blizzard.
What would you do?

_____

_____

Situation 4
While walking home in the pouring rain, you come to a stream that you usually walk across because it has stepping stones. However, the water is rising rapidly, and the current is much stronger than usual.
What would you do?

_____

Situation 5
Your room begins to shake, and you realize that an earthquake is taking place.
What would you do?

_____

_____

Activity 76

Applying Health Skills

Basic First Aid

A good way to be prepared for emergencies is to keep a well-stocked first aid kit in your home. Using the list of items at the right, complete the chart on the left to show the typical contents of a home first aid kit. Then answer the questions that follow.

Types of Items		small flashlight, tweezers, gauze pads, tissues, antiseptic ointment, thermometer, adhesive tape, scissors, cotton swabs, adhesive bandages, hand cleaner, activated charcoal, sterile eyewash, blanket, disposable gloves, syrup of ipecac, cold pack, plastic bags, triangular bandage, face mask
Dressings		
Instruments		
Equipment		
Medications		
Miscellaneous		

1. What is *first aid*?

_____

2. What are the universal precautions that help prevent the spread of disease through contaminated blood?

_____

_____

_____

3. What is a person's first responsibility in any emergency situation?

_____

4. What is the only situation in which a victim should be moved?

_____

Activity 77 — Applying Health Skills

Taking Care of Common Emergencies

You can effectively help someone who is hurt if you know how to give first aid in common emergencies. Read the list for each common emergency below. Check your knowledge by writing an *X* on the line in front of each item that tells what you should do.

Sprains

_____ Move the injured part to keep it from becoming stiff.

_____ Apply ice to reduce swelling and pain.

_____ Elevate the sprained part above the level of the heart.

First-Degree Burns

_____ Immerse the burned area in cold water, or apply cold compresses.

_____ Remove loose skin.

_____ Cover the burn with a sterile bandage.

Foreign Object in the Eye

_____ Lightly touch the object with a moistened cotton swab.

_____ Try to flush the object from the eye with clean water.

_____ Rub the eye vigorously.

Nosebleeds

_____ Have the person put his or her head down.

_____ Pinch the nose for 5 to 10 minutes.

_____ If bleeding continues, get medical help.

Insect Bites

_____ Wash the affected area.

_____ Apply a special lotion for bites.

_____ Leave the bite uncovered.

Poisoning

_____ Call the nearest poison control center.

_____ Induce vomiting in all cases.

_____ Read the label of anything the poison control center tells you to give the victim.

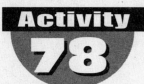

Applying Health Skills

Dealing with Life-Threatening Emergencies

   Listed below are the steps that should be taken in certain life-threatening emergencies. Put the steps in the order in which they should be done by writing the correct letter in the space at the left. The first one in each group has been done for you.

Saving a Choking Adult

_____ 1. Quickly thrust inward and upward, as if trying to lift the person.

_____ 2. Repeat thrusts until the food or object is dislodged.

_____ 3. Stand behind the person and wrap your arms around his or her waist.

_____ 4. Make a fist with one hand, and place it just above the person's navel.

Stopping Severe Bleeding

_____ 5. Apply direct pressure to the wound, using a clean cloth.

_____ 6. Apply pressure to the artery that supplies blood to the area of the wound.

_____ 7. Raise the site of bleeding above the level of the heart.

_____ 8. Have the person lie down.

Treating a Person in Shock

_____ 9. Have the person lie down and raise the feet higher than the head.

_____ 10. Look for signs of shock, such as a weak, rapid pulse and shallow breathing.

_____ 11. Cover the person with a blanket or coat to keep him or her warm.

_____ 12. Loosen tight clothing.

Giving CPR to Adults

_____ 13. Find a spot on lower half of the victim's breastbone.

_____ 14. Lock elbows, press down firmly on chest, and then release.

_____ 15. Place the heel of one hand on the spot located on the breastbone.

_____ 16. Give 15 chest compressions, pause and give 2 rescue breaths, then repeat.

Chapter **19** Health Inventory

Better Safe Than Sorry

Here is a handy checklist to help you act wisely in an emergency. In the space at the left, put a check next to each statement that describes you or your home.

_____ 1. A list of important telephone numbers is kept near the telephone.

_____ 2. I know the basic steps to follow when someone needs first aid.

_____ 3. Chemicals and cleaners are clearly marked and kept out of the reach of children.

_____ 4. The stairs and hallways in my home are kept clear and well lighted.

_____ 5. I use electrical appliances according to the manufacturers' directions.

_____ 6. I know how to control severe bleeding.

_____ 7. My home has working smoke alarms.

_____ 8. I know how to assess circulation to determine whether CPR is needed.

_____ 9. My family has an established escape plan in case of fire.

_____ 10. A well-stocked first aid kit is available in my home.

_____ 11. I never pull a plug by the cord.

_____ 12. I have a buddy with me when I do activities outdoors.

_____ 13. I never put my friends' feelings ahead of my own safety.

_____ 14. I use appropriate safety gear for sports activities.

_____ 15. I cross streets at crosswalks and obey traffic lights.

Score yourself:

Write the number of checks here.

12–15: Congratulations! Your safety rating is excellent!

8–11: Your safety rating is good, but you could improve.

Fewer than 8: You need to think about what you can do to raise your safety rating. Better safe than sorry.

Chapter 20 Study Guide

As you read the chapter, answer the following questions. Later you can use this guide to review the information in the chapter.

Lesson 1

1. List five factors that are part of your environment.

_____

_____

2. Identify the major sources of air pollution.

_____

_____

3. Name three damaging environmental consequences linked to air pollution.

_____

_____

4. Explain how the greenhouse effect contributes to global warming.

_____

_____

_____

5. Identify two ways in which water pollution can affect human health.

_____

_____

_____

6. Define *hazardous wastes*.

_____

7. Give three examples of common hazardous wastes.

_____

Lesson 2

8. Identify the three *R*s that people can follow to help clean up and protect the environment.

_____

_____

9. List two ways to help keep the air cleaner.

_____

_____

10. Define *nonrenewable resources*, and give an example of such a resource.

_____

11. List three ways to save water at home.

_____

_____

_____

12. Identify three kinds of objects that can be recycled.

_____

13. Identify three basic guidelines for precycling.

_____

_____

14. List three ways you can help others understand the importance of becoming involved in protecting the environment.

_____

_____

Activity 79

Applying Health Skills

Analyzing Pollution Sources

Complete the chart below to list the sources of air and water pollution and their negative effects on health. Then answer the questions.

Pollution	Air	Water
sources		
components		
negative effects		

1. What is one alternative to burying trash in landfills? What are its drawbacks?

_____

_____

_____

2. What should you do when you need to dispose of hazardous materials?

_____

_____

_____

Activity 80

Applying Health Skills

Surveying Recyclables

Some people do not realize how many items in their environment are recyclable. Complete the chart below by first looking around your classroom and listing one or two items that fit each category. Do the same at home. Then answer the questions.

Material	Classroom	Home
paper/ paperboard		
glass		
plastics		
aluminum		

1. What are the benefits of recycling?

_____

_____

2. What are some ways you could be a more environmentally conscious consumer?

_____

_____

_____

_____

Chapter 20 Health Inventory

How Can You Help the Environment?

Rate your awareness of environmental problems and what you can do to help. For each item below, circle the word that tells how often you behave as described.

always   sometimes   never   **1.** Rather than ride in a car, I walk or ride a bike.

always   sometimes   never   **2.** I turn off lights, radios, and television sets when I am not using them.

always   sometimes   never   **3.** I turn down the heat when no one is home.

always   sometimes   never   **4.** I do not run the dishwasher or washing machine unless I have a full load.

always   sometimes   never   **5.** I do not waste water by leaving it running.

always   sometimes   never   **6.** I bring a cloth or reusable plastic bag to carry my purchases when I go to the store.

always   sometimes   never   **7.** I use biodegradable detergents and other products.

always   sometimes   never   **8.** I help recycle paper, plastic, aluminum, and glass.

always   sometimes   never   **9.** I am willing to volunteer my time to make the environment cleaner and safer.

always   sometimes   never   **10.** I reuse items by repairing them, selling them, or donating them to charity.

always   sometimes   never   **11.** I choose products in reusable or recyclable packages.

always   sometimes   never   **12.** I use public transportation whenever necessary.

always   sometimes   never   **13.** I buy in bulk when I can.

always   sometimes   never   **14.** I use reusable materials instead of paper plates and cups.

Score yourself:

Give yourself 3 points for each *always* answer, 1 point for each *sometimes* answer, and 0 for each *never*. Write your score here.

36–42: Excellent; you are doing your part for a healthy environment.

26–35: Good; you are trying. Keep up the effort.

Fewer than 26: You need to do a better job of protecting the environment. See what you can do to improve. This is the only world we get.